Happily Ever After

My Journey with Guillain-Barré Syndrome and How I Got My Life Back

HOLLY GERLACH

Order this book online at www.trafford.com
or email orders@trafford.com

Most Trafford titles are also available at major online book retailers.

Printed in the United States of America.

ISBN: 978-1-4669-5380-2 (sc)
ISBN: 978-1-4669-5382-6 (hc)
ISBN: 978-1-4669-5381-9 (e)

Library of Congress Control Number: 2012915103

Trafford rev. 10/04/2012

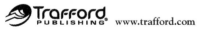 www.trafford.com

North America & international
toll-free: 1 888 232 4444 (USA & Canada)
phone: 250 383 6864 • fax: 812 355 4082

Contents

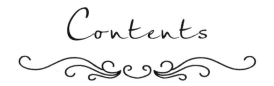

This book was made possible because of my mother who documented my progress every single day in a journal and because of my husband who helped fill in the blanks along the way

The names of friends, nurses, doctors, and hospitals have not been used, in respect of those who wish to remain anonymous

To my husband James, for being an amazing husband and father
My daughter Casey, for being my little angel
My mom Marilyn, for being at my side every step of the way
My family and friends, for supporting me when I needed them most
The nurses, doctors, therapists, and many others who helped get me
to where I am today
And all the complete strangers, who kept me in their prayers

Prelude

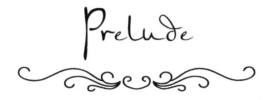

From the time I was old enough to know what a family was, it was something I couldn't wait to have. Maybe it was because I came from a divorced family that I longed for it that much more. I knew that I was destined to become a wife and mother since I was three years old. I dreamed about getting married, what the wedding would look like, what my husband would be like, and what our babies would look like throughout most of my childhood. In my young mind, I pictured getting married by twenty-five and starting a family by twenty-seven. I wanted the fairy-tale story, complete with my prince, our babies, and a happy ending.

When I grew up, at the age of twenty-four, on September 19, 2009, I married my best friend, James. I had my fairy-tale wedding surrounded by our closest friends and family. Of course, I immediately couldn't wait to start a family together.

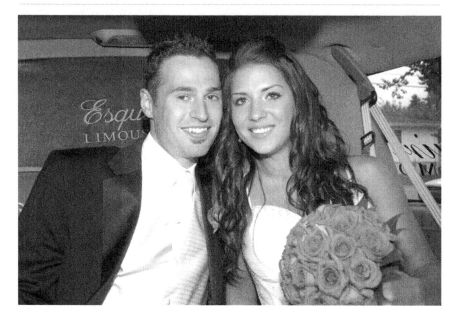

James and me on our wedding day

The following year, on May 19, 2010, we found out that we were expecting our first child together. I couldn't have been any happier; for all my dreams were coming true.

January 2011

On January 26, after nine months of an extremely enjoyable and pleasant pregnancy, I gave birth to our daughter Casey Marie. James and I had been together since we were eighteen years old, so it had been just the two of us for over eight years. But we were beyond excited with our new addition to the family.

James took a few weeks off from work to be home with Casey and me, and we spent those weeks adjusting to our new roles as parents. Parenthood felt very natural to both of us, and we absolutely loved our little family.

Casey was a little angel from day one. She immediately caught onto breastfeeding without any problems, rarely cried, and only woke up a couple of times in the night to nurse. She was such a happy and easygoing baby from day one and she brought great joy into our lives and everyone's around her.

I felt like the luckiest girl in the world. I had an amazing husband and a beautiful baby girl. My life was absolutely perfect.

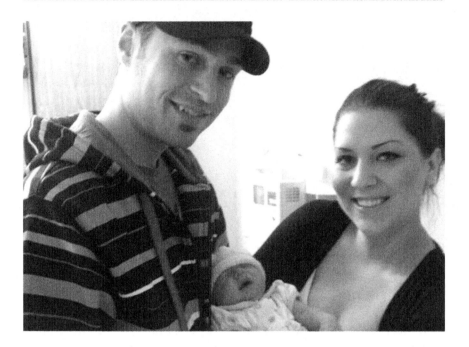

James, Casey and me

February

It was the evening before James was set to return to work after taking his paternity leave. Casey was almost three weeks old.

We were sitting on the couch videotaping Casey, who was starting to hold her head up on her own. We sent the video to my mom, who was in Toronto on business.

I remember that I noticed one of my fingertips was a little numb and tingly, but I didn't think anything of it. It kind of felt like the tingling when you burn yourself, and I figured that I must have burnt myself on something earlier and didn't pay any more attention to it.

Later, I started to feel really tired and weak and thought I must be getting the flu again (I had just gotten over it the week before). But pretty quickly, my weakness got worse; I was absolutely exhausted. My neck also started to hurt pretty badly, so I knew it couldn't be the flu.

As the neck pain worsened, James massaged my neck while I googled my symptoms on the Internet. Most of the sites I looked at suggested that I had a pinched nerve. James reminded me of the pinched nerve he had a few years back and said that it had caused him a lot of pain and weakness too, so it was probably that. I tried to just let it go, but after a few hours, the pain was way worse, and painkillers weren't helping at all. I decided to go to the medi-centre and see if they could give me something for the pain. I pumped a bottle for James to feed Casey, as I was breastfeeding and she was still nursing every couple of hours.

At the medi-center, I told the doctor that I thought I had a pinched nerve and described the pain in my neck and weakness in my legs. He looked me over and agreed that's probably what it was. He gave me a prescription for medication for the pain and wrote a referral to see a physiotherapist for the pinched nerve. As I left the doctor's office, I struggled down the hallway for my legs felt like rubber, as if they were going to give out on me. I remember being disappointed that the doctor couldn't fix me right then and there. But I figured the physiotherapist would fix me tomorrow. I went home, took some painkillers, and went to sleep.

I woke up about an hour later; I was in too much pain to sleep. My neck was aching so badly. I spent the next hour or two on my phone looking up massages and stretches on YouTube that relieved pinched nerves. But no matter what I did, nothing helped.

Around three o'clock in the morning, Casey woke up to nurse. I stood up and fell to my knees as my legs buckled and completely gave out on me. James woke up, asked if I was OK, and I told him no. I couldn't take the pain anymore and told him to take me to the hospital. I figured that at the emergency room, they could at least give me something stronger for the pain until I could see a physiotherapist. James had to be at work in less than four hours, and I also didn't want to bring my newborn into the emergency room, so I again pumped a couple of bottles for James and had him drop me off at the hospital. I figured that it would take me no more than a few hours and that I would be home in time to take care of Casey when James went to work.

I only waited for half an hour in the emergency room when they brought me into the triage room. I was happy that things were moving so quickly because my cell phone died right when I got to the hospital, and I didn't have anything to keep me occupied. The hospital staff took my vitals and some blood and had me wait for the doctor. I watched people coming in that were ten times sicker than I looked, and I started to feel guilty for coming in for a pinched nerve.

The doctor saw me around 4:30 a.m. and looked me over. He immediately informed me that he didn't think it was a pinched nerve and that he wanted to review my blood work when it came back. He gave me something for the pain, and it took the edge off enough for me to doze off in my chair.

Around 5:30 a.m., my blood work came back, and the doctor said he wanted to have a neurologist come down and see me. I was nervous, but a part of me was intrigued by what could be going on with me. Nothing like this had ever happened to me. Since I was a little girl, I had generally been very healthy, and other than just having a baby, I hadn't been in the hospital for any long period of time.

At this point, I asked to use the phone, and I called James. I told him about how a neurologist was going to come down and see me and that he had no choice but to stay home from work to be with with Casey until I got home. I knew that it would be a hard phone call, considering that it was his first day back from work in over three weeks.

He was going to run out of bottles of breast milk soon, so I told him to use the tin of formula we had on hand just in case, until I was home. I was disappointed as I had wanted to strictly breastfeed Casey, and I hoped the switch to formula and then back to breast milk didn't confuse her. After our phone call, I went back to my chair and waited.

Around 7:00 a.m., the neurologist still hadn't come down, but the nurses moved me out of the triage room and into a private area full of comfy leather recliners. I was the only person in the room, and I leaned back in my chair and slept for over an hour.

The neurologist finally arrived just after eight. He didn't say much. He told me to squeeze his hands and then he tested my knee and elbow reflexes. To me, everything felt completely normal. But it wasn't. He said my strength was weaker than it should be and that I had no reflexes in my legs or arms. He said he thought he knew what was wrong with me but wanted me to have some tests done before he could confirm anything. I asked him what he thought it was, and he said he would give me more details about it if that's what it turned out to be.

I asked the nurse for permission to use the phone again, and she brought me to a lounge that had a phone in it. The weakness in my legs was getting worse, and I struggled to walk there. I had to use the railings on the side of the walls to hold myself up. I called James and told him that they might know what it was but that they wouldn't confirm it until they knew for sure. James didn't think that was a good sign. I was pretty confident that I was fine and that everything would be fixed soon. James wanted to come to the hospital, but I really didn't want Casey to be around all the hospital germs, so I told him to stay at home and that I would be home in a few hours.

I was admitted into the emergency room around 9:00 a.m. on February 22, and given my own room where I waited to have my first tests, which were x-rays. As I was rolled down the hall in a wheelchair to have my x-rays done, I saw several people that looked very sick. I felt so out of place as I really didn't look like anything was wrong with me. And by this point, with the medication they had given me, the pain was way better, so other than being very tired and weak, I really didn't feel that bad.

After the x-rays, I waited back in my room and slept. When I woke up to use the washroom, I could hardly stand anymore. My legs were so weak and flimsy that the nurses got me a wheelchair and helped me use the washroom. Then I went back to my room and slept some more.

The neurologist came back a few hours later, around noon, and told me that I needed to have a spinal tap done. They needed to remove some spinal fluid to confirm his theory. He started to explain the process of removing the fluid from my spine, when I told him that I had just had a baby three weeks before. I had been given an epidural, so I was familiar with the process. They prepped me for the procedure, and it went off smoothly. Just like the epidural, I barely felt it.

Afterward, I again slept some more. Then around three in the afternoon, the doctor came in and told me what he thought it was that I had. It was Guillain-Barré syndrome, or GBS. He told me that it was a very rare autoimmune disorder that hit about one in a million people. It is defined by the fast onset of weakness, which is accompanied by tingling, pain, and paralysis. Basically, my immune system was attacking my nervous system. I would need to be admitted into the hospital and monitored to see how severe things got because the illness could vary in severity. No one is certain what causes GBS, but many cases are reported within a few weeks after another illness such as a cold or the flu. Other cases have been reported a few weeks after pregnancy or birth, and some after a major surgery. In my case, I had had all three: the flu about a week before, a baby, and a C-section.

I could tell by how my body felt that there was no way I could even get up anymore, so I asked him to bring me a phone to use. I called James and told him that he needed to come in. I then called my mom in Toronto and told her I was in the hospital, that the doctors thought I had a serious illness, and that she needed to come back to Edmonton. She made arrangements for the first available flight home.

The next few hours are a blur, probably from a lack of sleep. I don't have any recollection of being moved, but I was admitted to the Stroke and Neurology ward on the fifth floor. James and Casey came shortly after, and I resumed breastfeeding my daughter. I slept on and off for the rest of the evening. My mom got there around midnight. The nurses were extremely accommodating; they brought in a bassinet from Labor and Delivery for Casey and also an electric breast pump so that I could pump and someone else could feed her.

James had brought me my phone charger, and I was able to use my phone again. I remember texting my friends and telling them what I knew so far. Everyone was scared for me, and my girlfriends that lived out of town felt especially helpless. One of my best friends was out of town for a job interview to work on a cruise ship, and she learned of my situation just before her interview. I'm sure it took everything she had to keep it together during that interview.

I also remember going on Facebook and saying I felt like I was on an episode of House. The doctors hadn't confirmed that I had GBS for sure, and I felt like a patient on House that the doctors had no clue how to fix. My pain was starting to worsen again, but now, instead of just my neck, it was also in my back and all over my skin. My skin was suddenly so sensitive that whenever anyone barely touched me, I would scream in pain. I was given more medication, but it didn't help at all. I was told by the nurses and doctors that I needed to stop breastfeeding because the medication I was receiving could be harmful to Casey. So we switched over to formula right away.

I remember wanting to get up to go to the bathroom, but I could barely move my body. So I had to use a bedpan. When they rolled me over to place it under me, I screamed in pain. My muscles were so tight that even the slightest bend in my knees left me screaming and crying. Every time I had to pee, they would have to put the bedpan under me, and I would cry and scream. The nurses eventually started log rolling me instead of bending my knee, which wasn't as painful.

The results from my spinal tap weren't back yet, so the next morning, I had an MRI done on my brain to rule out any other conditions. My mom came with me, and I was pretty nervous as I didn't know what to expect.

They rolled my bed into the lab, and when I saw the MRI machine, I couldn't believe how small it was. I was expecting it to be a lot bigger, and I started to panic. I have been extremely claustrophobic since I was little, and I knew that I would not do well in the machine. I was given goggles so that I would only see black instead of the walls of the tunnel. The goggles also had a radio station with music playing to help keep me occupied. Then I was given a button to push if, for some reason, I needed to come out of the machine.

Once I was in, it was very loud, hot, and scary. I started freaking out within a few seconds; I tried to listen to the music, but I just couldn't stop thinking about it. I started to have a panic attack and felt like I couldn't breathe. I pressed the button and was brought back out of the machine. The man operating the MRI machine asked me why had I pressed the button, and I told him I was very claustrophobic and couldn't handle it. To me, he seemed annoyed. He said it was only for two minutes and that I needed to get this test done. I once again went back into the machine and once again started panicking. I tried to take deep breaths and started counting. It didn't help. I pressed the button again, was brought out, and I asked how much longer it would be. He said thirty seconds. So for the last thirty seconds, I breathed as deeply as I could and counted and listened to the music. By the time it was done, I was bawling. We went back to my room, and I prayed to God that I would never have to undergo that again.

That evening, another neurologist came to see me. This one had had quite a bit of experience with Guillain-Barré syndrome. The test results from my spinal tap had come back, and it was at this point that I was diagnosed with Guillain-Barré syndrome. The bad news was that there was no cure. The good news was that once patients hit their absolute worst (plateau), they would start improving and most often make a complete full recovery. He told me there were different degrees of GBS. Patients with very mild cases could be better and return home in a week, whereas patients with more severe cases could get to the point where they would be completely paralysed and eventually need to learn how to walk again. In those cases, recovery could take anywhere from six months to several years. I remember thinking there was no way that would be me. I still thought I would be out in a few days.

The doctor told me that because of how quick and debilitating the illness was, many people feel suicidal at some point. I was in so much pain that I was already there. It was the most excruciating pain I had ever gone through in my life (and let's not forget that I had gone through twelve hours of labor just weeks before), and I already didn't think I could take much longer of this.

He decided to start me on medication for the treatment of GBS. It wouldn't cure me, but it would hopefully speed up my recovery. It was called intravenous immunoglobulin (IVIG), a process that involved pumping healthy blood into my body intravenously over five days. Its purpose was to supply my body with healthy antibodies found in blood, which would help neutralize the harmful antibodies in my blood. I asked the doctor how they would know if the IVIG was working, and he told me that I would start to regain my strength and slowly get stronger. I was so relieved and hopeful. I couldn't wait to start getting stronger. They started me on the treatment, although looking back now, I have no recollection of it.

That night, while I slept, my mom noticed that my breathing was slowing down. Sometimes, I wouldn't take a breath for a few seconds. She notified the nurses, who told her that it could be a sign that my diaphragm was weakening as well and that I could go into respiratory failure. If that were to happen, I would need to be transferred to the intensive care unit (ICU) to be put on a ventilator. They said they would monitor me overnight and see if I improved in the morning.

The following day, my breathing was better, but the doctor still decided to notify the ICU just in case.

My body, however, was still getting worse. I was getting weaker and weaker and was in even more pain. My mom and stepdad went to the store to pick up a few things, and they hadn't even been gone ten minutes when they received a call from James that my breathing had deteriorated in the short time that they were gone and that I was being transferred to the ICU immediately. The doctors also decided to stop the IVIG treatment. They wanted to start me on plasmapheresis, another treatment for GBS. This process involved removing the blood from my body through a catheter, pumping it into a machine that removed the harmful antibodies, and then again pumping it back into my body. Once I was transferred to the ICU, I would begin the plasmapheresis treatment.

I was transferred to the ICU in the early afternoon on February 24, *Day 3* in the hospital. In order to administer the plasmapheresis, a catheter tube would need to be inserted into a large vein in my groin on the upper right hand side of my thigh. My family waited in the waiting room, and once the catheter was inserted and I was all settled in my room, they would be allowed to see me.

Several hospital staff came in for the procedure. It's funny the things I remember. I barely remember any of my nurses up until this point, but I remember the nurse that was in the room that day with me perfectly. She was the first nurse that seemed to really care about me. She was so comforting and rubbed my forehead while I lay there in pain.

I watched as one of the doctors reached down to where they were inserting the catheter in my thigh, and the pain hit me like a brick. I literally felt like someone's entire fist was in a gaping wound in my thigh. For all I know, it was. I started screaming for medication, and my nurse said that they would get me something very shortly. I was hysterical. The pain was unbearable, and I was sure I was going to pass out at any minute.

The doctor left the room and came back with another doctor, who started to feel around the incision, and again, it felt like the doctor was putting his entire hand in my thigh. I was screaming at the top of my lungs and begging for them to please just get me something for the pain because I just couldn't handle it.

The doctors left again, and the nurse rubbed my forehead. She told me I was going to be OK and tried to calm me down. I kept crying for what seemed like forever, and after what felt like ten minutes, although I'm sure it was probably not even one, I was given something for the pain.

The next thing I remember, I was being wheeled down the hallway into another room. It was very bright in the room, and there was a ton of hospital staff everywhere. It reminded me a lot of the room where I had an emergency C-section with Casey. I was transferred onto a table, and I think it was at this moment that I realized I was now in an operating room.

My family patiently waited for me to be finished with the catheter placement when a nurse came and asked them if the doctor had been out to see them yet. They said no, and she said she would get him right away. The doctor showed up a few minutes later. He started off by apologizing, and basically said they had screwed up. While they were trying to insert the catheter into my vein, my femoral artery had been punctured, and I was bleeding internally. They would need to do emergency surgery that could take several hours. They didn't know if I would make it through the surgery.

My family was not expecting this and sat there in shock. My mom tried to hold it together, but she couldn't. She started bawling and had to rush out of the room to throw up. While in the bathroom, she prayed and said, "Please, God, don't take her from me."

James called his parents, and when he tried to tell them what was going on, he couldn't even speak. He started to tell his parents what was happening and started crying. He was so scared of losing me. My family started making phone calls, and all our closest friends started rushing to the hospital.

I don't recall waking up, but I've been told that I was in a great mood. The surgery was a success, so of course I had every reason to be, but considering what I woke up to, I'm still shocked that I didn't completely freak out. I had a large breathing tube in my mouth and down my throat to help me breathe, so I could no longer talk. In my nose was a smaller tube, called a nasogastric tube (NG tube), which was how I would be fed until I was off the breathing tube. I had four catheters, one in my jugular on the right side of my neck as well as my left inner thigh to administer the plasmapheresis, one in the vein in my right arm to administer my medications (called a PICC line), and one in my urethra to drain the urine from my bladder. My paralysis had also worsened, and I could no longer move my legs at all.

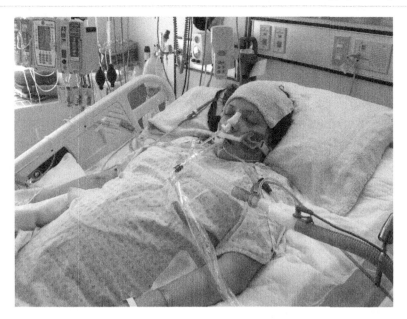

First photo of me in the hospital

Even though I was so drowsy and out of it, when I saw my best friend back in the city from her interview on the cruise ship, I was actually able to mouth the words, "How did it go?" She was very proud to let me know that she had gotten the job, and I remember being extremely proud of her.

The second day after the surgery, *Day 4*, I continued to deteriorate even more. I started to give up hope, and my mood drastically changed. When GBS attacks the nervous system, although it destroys the nerve sheath, which was causing my paralysis, I could still feel sensations. Not only could I feel them, but also everything was hypersensitive, and the slightest touch was painful. I was in so much pain, both in my neck and back and all over my skin. I was on so many medications for the pain that I was completely out of it. I was surrounded by my closest friends and family, and I came to the conclusion that I was dying.

I called my mom over to me and mouthed the words, "Just let me go." She started crying and told me that she promised I would get better, but that it would just take time. I needed to hold on. I wouldn't listen. I just kept mouthing the words while crying, "Just let me go, Mom. I'm ready to go."

I know that the only reason why I managed to keep going was because I had my family with me at all times. James took a temporary leave of absence from work to take care of Casey, so they were at the hospital all day and every day with me. And along with friends and family visiting constantly, I was rarely alone. Anytime I was alone, I would start to have a panic attack, so the hospital brought in a pull-out chair for my mom to sleep in so she could stay overnight. She stayed with me almost every single night I was in the hospital, and once a week, James and Casey would stay. I was lucky enough that my mom mostly works from home and that, other than a few meetings a week, she was there with me the entire time.

The hospital also transformed a waiting room into my own personal family room. Many times, we would have too many visitors at once, and it was nice that they would have somewhere to go and hang out. My family turned it into their own little area, with my dad bringing in a coat rack for their jackets and a bookcase to stack things on.

Word traveled fast, and the support began pouring in. Day after day, I had someone new coming to visit me, from my closest friends to people that I hadn't seen in years. A woman that had GBS before even came to see me and let me know that I would get through this.

Some people would bring in food for my family while at the hospital, which was fantastic as many times they would simply forget to eat. Everyone reacted to seeing me differently, but the men seemed to be the most bothered by it. Several of my closest guy friends couldn't keep it together and cried, and they left the room when they saw me for the first time. I could definitely understand why. Between all the tubes, and how terrible I looked, it must have been extremely difficult. But what made it even harder on my visitors was that I couldn't talk to them. I know they were just waiting for me to tell them that I was OK, but all I could do was mouth words. This made for many one-sided conversations and many awkward silences.

Unfortunately for my visitors, this was also the week that was minus thirty outside. The GBS was affecting my autonomic nervous system as well, meaning that it was changing my blood pressure, my heart rate, and my body temperature. I was so hot all the time. I felt like my room was over fifty degrees and that I was going to faint at any moment. I remember my family putting cold cloths on my forehead over and over and over again.

I was lucky that there was at least a thermostat in my room and that my family was able to turn it down as low as they could. To me, the room felt warm, but it was freezing. Whenever someone would come to visit me, they would stay in their winter jackets. My mom brought in blankets for people to use, and one of my more amusing memories was when my brother stayed overnight with me and had to wear my mom's fur jacket and mitts all night long. One of my girlfriends, who always has very cold hands, also came in very handy as it was instant relief for her to put her cold hands on my forehead.

Those first few weeks, I was hot the majority of the time and then, on top of that, I would have hot flashes that would leave me struggling to catch my breath as I almost fainted. For the majority of the time, I had a cold cloth on my forehead to keep me cool, and when it got worse, my family would pat my face and legs with another cold cloth.

Since I couldn't talk anymore, I quickly struggled to communicate with my family and friends. The hospital brought in a communication board with letters for me to point to so I could spell out words and short sentences. It took a long time to spell out each word, and I was frustrated many times, but at least it worked. I was able to connect with people in some way.

Because many of my symptoms were recurring, I found myself spelling out the same phrases over and over again. My family and I agreed on specific movements that would represent what I wanted, and James drew pictures that could be explained to new visitors and nurses of what I wanted. I would open my mouth and shake my head when I was in pain and needed more medication. If I looked up and down, I was hot and needed a cold cloth patted on my face and legs. If I "keyboarded" my fingers, I wanted the communication board to spell something out. And if I was wiggling my arms, I needed to be repositioned to help with stiff muscles. Even though I couldn't move my legs, I could still feel everything, and I was getting very sore.

Even with everything going on around me, I somehow managed to keep my sense of humor. After having been seen by one of the more "attractive" doctors, I spent a very long time pointing to letters and spelling out the words "Hot Doctor" to my girlfriends. Another time, after having a nurse that just didn't seem concerned with my pain at all, I spelt out the word "Evil" to my dad, with a smile on my face. I think it was times like these that reminded my family that I was still the same Holly, even if it didn't seem like it at all.

The plasmapheresis was given over six days and took a few hours at a time. I don't actually remember the procedure, but I remember being in even more pain whenever the procedure was administered to me. My family later told me that it was because I was told not to move an inch. I often moved my torso around in bed to relieve the pain caused by lying down for long periods of time, so keeping still was extremely uncomfortable. I also still had excruciating pain in my neck and back that rarely went away.

Sometimes the pain in my back was almost unbearable, and I would have family members massage me for hours on end. This was extremely difficult; I was stuck on my back so they had to massage me from underneath my back. I was given a prescription for a medicated lotion to help with inflammation, and I'm sure we went through a bottle a day. I quickly made my favourites and communicated to my family that James was the best massager and that my mom "sucked." I'm sure my mom was partly happy as this meant that James and other family members with strong hands ended up massaging me a lot more often. My mom must still have had plenty of practice, because as the weeks went on, she improved drastically.

James asked me if I wanted to see the incisions from my emergency surgery. I did, so he took a picture with his phone. When I saw the picture, I couldn't believe I was looking at my own body. I had a three-inch scar on the right hand side of my inner thigh that went up toward my pelvis. But the other one was way worse. It was a very long and thick black line all the way down my stomach. It was about six inches long, starting at the bottom of my rib cage going down to the top of my pubic bone. There were also about thirty-five staples keeping the incision closed. I had literally been cut in half.

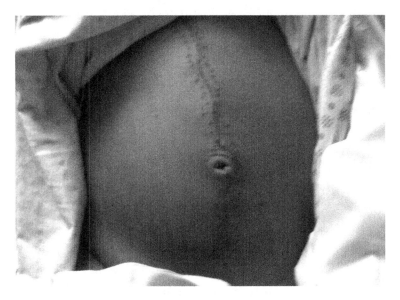

One of my scars from the surgery

I was devastated. After I had my C-section, I was so happy with how tiny the scar was; it was almost invisible. And now I would have this ugly huge scar on my body for the rest of my life.

When I look back on those first two weeks, I really don't remember all that much. I have a few short memories, but even with some of those, I wonder if I only remember being told about them. I was very heavily medicated, so most of the time I was either sleeping or dazed.

I hallucinated often, although I only know that now—I didn't know that at the time. It all seemed real to me. First off, I constantly felt like I was in different hospital rooms throughout the ICU. I thought I was in one room when my artery was ruptured and then in another when I was administered my plasmapheresis. I thought I was in one room during the day and then in a different room at night. But I wasn't. I was in the same room every day, all the time.

Even though I couldn't move my legs, I would sometimes think they were moving on their own. It would feel like my legs were floating, and sometimes I even thought I was floating right off my bed when I clearly wasn't. My brother said I told him my leg fell off the bed once, and he had to convince me that it hadn't moved.

In the middle of the night, I panicked over the balloons in my room as I thought they were a group of people standing in the corner. I freaked out over a jar sitting on the counter as I was convinced that there was a human skull in the jar.

Once I woke up in a panic, screaming and crying, and when my mom finally calmed me down, I told her I had dreamed that cats were eating me.

I also had so many visitors during those first few weeks that sometimes I would ask my family if they had really come or if I had just dreamed that they had. At other times, James would talk about the people that had come to visit me, but I had no recollection of them even being there. I didn't know what was real and what wasn't. Things felt backward; when I slept, I would dream about living my normal life, and when I was awake, I was living a nightmare.

March

In the first few days of March, the plasmapheresis finished. It was such a long and painful experience, and we were all relieved to be done with it. However, I was still unable to breathe on my own without the help of a ventilator, and it looked like it would be a long time before I could come off it.

The doctors suggested the removal of the breathing tube and insertion of a tracheostomy or "trach" tube instead. The tracheotomy would be performed by making an incision in my "stoma," or windpipe, through my neck and inserting the trach tube for me to breathe. The trach would be a lot more comfortable for me as I would no longer have a tube in my mouth, and my family would be able to see me smile. I would also be able to mouth words easier. I was very excited about the trach as I would also be able to speak for small periods of time when using a speaking valve.

On March 2, *Day 9*, I was anesthetized and the tracheotomy was performed right in my room. I don't recall waking up from this procedure either, but I remember the first time I had to breathe with it. The breaths felt different and were forced through me. Sometimes, the alarm would sound, and the nurses would tell me that I needed to take in a breath.

I also remember the first time my trach had to be suctioned. My tracheostomy tube would constantly fill up with lung secretions, which made it harder to breathe in. My trach would need to be suctioned by the respiratory therapists (RTs) to clear the tube of mucus so that I would be able to breathe in easier.

Suctioning was done by placing a plastic catheter down my trach and suctioning out any mucus I had. Whenever this was done, I would cough so badly that I wouldn't be able to breathe, and I thought I was going to die every time. And this happened several times an hour. It was hard for my family to watch; since I had no use of my vocal cords, no sound would be made when I coughed, so it simply looked like I was violently choking.

The RTs were amazing at calming me down and assured me that I would catch my breath once I was done coughing. And once I was done, I could breathe a lot easier than before.

Now that I no longer had the breathing tube down my throat, I was able to mouth out words without having to use the communication board as often. But for the most part, only James was able to read my lips, so unless he was around, we stuck with the board. Day after day, I would point to the letters on the board, and my family would write down the words on a whiteboard to spell out sentences. They were constantly losing the lid to the marker, so by spelling out the words, I told them to buy a marker with a click top that didn't have a lid. My family laughed; even though I was very out of it, I was still able to think up something that smart and communicate it to them.

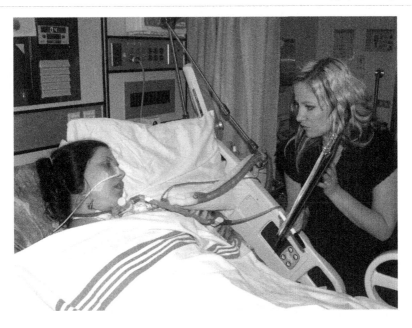

Using the communication board to talk with a friend

The board helped us all so much during the days, but at nighttime, since I could barely move or make a sound, I had no way to get my mom's attention if I needed something. I was so relieved when I figured out a way to click my tongue in my mouth that made a loud "cluck" sound. This would become my way of getting anyone's attention for the next few months.

With the way things were going, James made the decision to take paternity leave from his job. It was unclear how long I would be in the hospital for, and he would need to stay home with Casey until I was better. My family applied for disability insurance for me, but until I was approved, and until James' paternity insurance came in, neither of us had an income.

That's when our amazing friends stepped in. They knew that not only did we no longer have any income coming in in the meantime, we also had the added cost of formula since I could no longer breastfeed. Through the grapevine, and with the help of Facebook, they announced that they would be taking any form of donations for our family. People started donating things right away, such as diapers, formula, clothes, and money. We were completely amazed by the amount of support pouring in.

Now that I had the trach in, I was able to use the speaking valve that allowed me to talk for short periods of time. The speaking valve was a one-way valve that attached to the tracheostomy tube. When I breathed in, the valve would open, bringing air into the trach. Then when I breathed out, the valve closed and air would travel through my vocal cords, allowing sounds to be made.

The first time I used it, I couldn't quite make any sounds. It was hard to breathe in so quickly and talk while breathing out, but I eventually got it and managed to get a few words out. My voice was very quiet and sounded different as it was extremely hoarse, but James could still understand me. My first words in over a week were, "I sound scary." And even though I had been struggling to communicate during the last week, I couldn't think of anything else to say. I just kept repeating, "I don't know what to say." My mom sat by with the video camera and taped this huge milestone. It took a lot more work to breathe through the valve than just the trach, so I was winded very quickly, and I asked to be taken off the speaking valve after only a few minutes. But it was enough; my family was thrilled to finally hear my voice again.

About a week into March, I felt like I had woken up from a dream. The first thing I noticed was that I was no longer wearing my wedding ring. I felt sick to my stomach, thinking that I must have lost it somewhere since I had arrived. But James reassured me; they had removed it when I was admitted, and he had it in a safe place.

When I looked around my room, I saw posters full of our family photos everywhere. Pictures of Casey when she was born, pictures from our wedding day, and pictures of my family and friends surrounded me. Flowers weren't allowed in the ICU so everyone brought in *Get*

Well cards, and my mom had bordered the entire room with them. I remember thinking, "When did they put these up?" My mom had decorated the room with stickers and pink boas (my favourite color). I had no recollection of any of these being put up.

The RTs had also put up a poster they had made to track my breathing trials (the amount of minutes that I would try breathing completely on my own without the help of the ventilator). They named the poster Hollywood's Breathing Trials; they had come up with the theme of Hollywood for me, which couldn't have been more perfect as my nickname is Hollywood, and I have quite the obsession with celebrity gossip.

My mom brought in pink construction paper and cut out stars that she was going to put up around the room. Instead, I suggested that we write down my milestones on the stars and put them on the roof above my bed so I could look at them and see my progress. We made one for my first time on the speaking valve, and as I lay in bed staring up at it, I could only hope that there would be more stars to come.

Don't ask me why, but for some reason I thought of our bills. I was the one that paid them at home, and I panicked when I realized that it was past the first, when I regularly paid them. James brought in our online banking information, and instead of just having him do it, I insisted on having my mom help me navigate the online banking website on her laptop and paid the bills myself. I guess it made me feel like I was able to do something normal. I had completely lost the ability to do anything on my own, so it felt good for me to do this.

Because I wasn't moving my muscles, physical therapists fitted me for foot and hand splints to ensure that my muscles didn't stiffen up. The hand splints were made of a type of cast material that would keep my hand and fingers straight because, as my muscles stiffened and contracted from lack of movement, my fingers started to bend toward my body. The foot splints were foam boots that were used to stabilize my foot so that it wouldn't drop forward, which would cause problems with my ankle later on. I had to wear the splints on and off every few hours. To keep the rest of my joints flexible, my family was shown how to do range of motion exercises, which involved moving and stretching my limbs. Nurses or family and friends would take turns doing what we would call "Range" about three times a day.

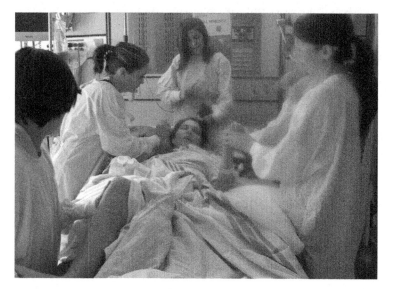

Range of Motion exercises

Twice a week, I had x-rays done on my chest to look at my lungs. Nurses would try and sit me up in my bed to place the x-ray board under my back, but the slightest bending of my back would send sharp pains shooting down through my thighs. I would scream as loud as I could, but because of the trach, no sound would come out. My mom would see me with my mouth wide open, crying in pain, and stop the nurses. They tried to move me slower, but it didn't help, and the pain was just as severe. It felt like when you bend your finger too far back, but here it was with my torso. I wouldn't let them try again so they would instead roll me over to place the board under my back. This was still extremely painful and I was left crying after it, but it was at least bearable.

One of my x-rays showed that the upper lobe of my left lung had collapsed. When a person is standing, the heart rests in front of the left lung. But when lying down, the heart rests on top of the lung. My heart was putting pressure on my lung twenty-four hours a day as I was lying in my hospital bed all day and night. The doctors wanted me to start sitting up in a recliner chair a few hours a day to take the pressure off my lung, but I was not in any position to be moved into a sling to lift me out of the bed. So until I improved a bit, they would keep watch over it and make sure it didn't get any worse.

I knew I had the most amazing friends and family, and even nurses, judging from the things they would do for me. Some of my friends came in with nail polish to paint my nails, and others came with tweezers to pluck my eyebrows. A few of the RTs even started painting my nails every week. I have always cared a lot about my appearance, and they knew that little things like that would make me feel better. I have really long hair, and it was starting to get matted in the back from constantly lying on it, so friends and family would spend hours combing and brushing out the knots. One day, one of my girlfriends even did my makeup. She was pregnant and going to have her baby any day, so it made my day that she could take the time to help me feel more like myself.

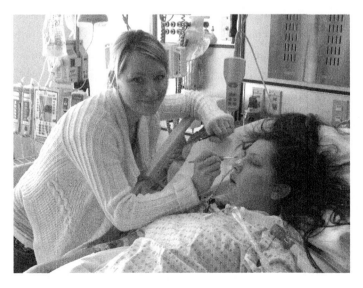

Getting my make-up done

It was very dry in my room, so my lips were extremely chapped, and people brought in all different kinds of lip balm for me. But they were so bad that they started peeling. My husband was fantastic; he would peel off the chunks of dry skin from my lips several times a day. It really lifted my spirits to be taken care of the way I was.

James even hooked up my iPod for me so that I could listen to my favorite music in my room, and one of my girlfriends downloaded the new Britney Spears album for me when it came out because she knew I would love it.

As the days went by, and the pain in my back worsened, the doctors doubled my medication. I was asking for meds so often that they decided that I needed a higher dose. I was on a strict schedule for the meds, but I was also allowed to have a top-up every hour when the pain was too hard to handle, and I remember watching the clock waiting until I was able to be given another dose. Then I would have my family call the nurse. Some days, I had top-ups every single hour all day long.

In the ICU, each nurse has only one patient, so they were always very quick to respond, but whenever they were busy and would take longer than a few minutes, I would get so angry very quickly and beg for a top-up. My family felt so helpless that they couldn't do more for me. I recall telling everyone that I couldn't handle the pain. I actually wanted to die. I never wanted to be alone in case I needed more meds because I had no way of getting the nurses' attention.

The doctors tried several different types of medication before they finally found one that seemed to help more than the others. They administered the top-ups by injecting it into the PICC line that was in the vein in my arm. Whenever they did so, it resulted in an instant high and instant pain relief. I felt like a drug addict.

The top-ups didn't last very long, so they gave me the option of having the medicine injected right into my skin on my stomach. It would take longer to start working, but the effects would last a lot longer than the top-ups. I tried it a few times, but it really did take too long to set in. Although the prick of the needle into my skin didn't hurt, when the medication surged into my body, it stung so badly. I pretty much took the top-ups only intravenously, which gave me almost instant relief as well a rush that I can't explain.

Although it had only been a couple of weeks, I felt like I had been in the hospital forever. Everyone said I would get better, but I wasn't. I was getting worse. My paralysis had now spread upward, so I could no longer move anything below my neck. I would try as hard as I could to move my hands, but they wouldn't move. Struggling to move my body when it wouldn't was painful, both emotionally and physically. Not being able to use my hands, I could no longer point to the letters on the communication board. My family had to point and I would nod when they picked the letters I wanted them to use.

My doctors assured me that once I had reached my plateau (hit my absolute worst), I would start to recover, and I would get better and better every day. It would just take time. I found it very hard to believe that I was ever going to make it through this. I found myself praying that I would just die.

My doctors and nurses could see in my eyes that I was giving up hope, so one staff member came up with an idea. They had had a patient in the ICU that had GBS a couple of years before; his condition was just as severe as mine was, and he had completely recovered. They thought that, maybe if he came in to see me, it would show me that people with this disease do recover, but that it would just take time and to not give up hope.

They asked me if it was OK to share my story with him, and they would get in touch with him and ask him if he would come to see me and share his story with me. He was beyond willing to come in and share his struggle with me and hoped that it would help. It wasn't long before the meeting was set up, and he came to the hospital to visit me on *Day 14.*

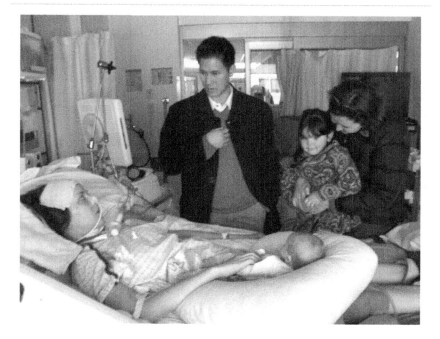

Meeting a previous GBS survivor and his family

So far, our cases were very similar; we had both deteriorated very quickly and were put on ventilators around the same time. Oddly enough, I was even in the same room in the ICU that he had been in for about four months. Hearing that he was there for that long terrified me, but seeing him standing by my bedside, looking like a completely normal and healthy person, made me feel a lot better. He was definitely an inspiration.

My mom would play the song, "The Climb" by Miley Cyrus over and over on my iPod. It is a song about someone getting through a rough time. Whenever I listened to it, I cried my eyes out. I just wanted this all to be over. The song made me think of him, and for a moment I thought that if he could get through this, I could too.

A few days later, the nausea started. I felt sick, but I couldn't throw up. I think my nausea was because of all the different medications I was on. The mix of everything in my stomach felt like too much. Even the thought of being given meds made me sick to my stomach. The nausea seemed to come out of nowhere, but now that it was here, it rarely went away.

The doctors switched every week, so every time I had a new doctor, they would suggest a new medication to treat the nausea. Sometimes they worked but usually only temporarily. Sometimes nothing worked. I just wanted to feel normal again. I remember asking James to bring me marijuana. I knew that was something that I'd used before to treat nausea, and I knew that it would work. James tried not to laugh and told me he could not bring me marijuana.

The nausea would come and go throughout the day, but some days were worse than others. I hated being around people when I felt this way. So other than my parents, James' parents, and our very closest friends, my visitors stopped coming as often. No one knew if I would be having a good day or a bad day, and I constantly turned people away.

But every morning, James would come in with Casey. I could hear when they were coming down the hallway to my room because all the nurses would start "oohing" and "aahing" over her. The nurses in other rooms would come out to see the two of them. They all loved her from the beginning. She was only a few weeks old, and she quickly became well known around the unit.

It became a daily thing for me to wonder what new thing she would be wearing, and I couldn't wait to see her. People were donating clothes to us by the boxful, so every day James would dress her up in a new adorable outfit. We still had the bassinet from labor and delivery in my room so that's where Casey spent a large part of her time. We were so lucky to have such a great baby, as she would spend hours in her bassinet completely content and barely ever making a peep. James and my brother would watch hockey, and I remember watching Casey as she stared at the TV. She was a hockey fan already.

The nurses would often come into my room so they could hold Casey. James always had such a hard time letting other people hold her, and he quickly became known as the "Baby Hog." But I later learned, with me in the shape I was in, that he felt like Casey was all he had left. He felt that he needed to do everything in his power to protect that little girl, which was why he always wanted to keep her within arm's reach.

James and my mom wanted to keep Casey as connected to me as possible, so they would try putting her on my bed with me, but a lot of the time I would say no. It devastated me that even though she was lying in my bed with me, I couldn't reach out and touch her or hold her in my arms. I was in so much pain whenever anyone barely touched me that I was afraid that even her tiny movements would hurt me or make me nauseous.

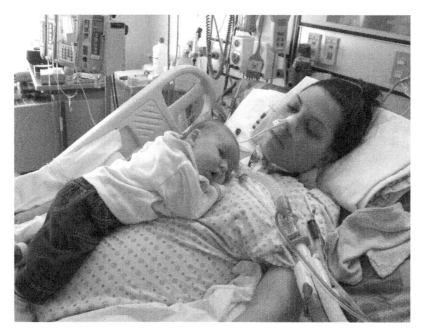

Cuddling with Casey

I think a lot of people thought that I had postpartum depression as I seemed uninterested in my baby, but I truly believe that I didn't. I was dealing with this devastating illness, and it broke my heart that I couldn't be the mom that she needed me to be. She was only a little over a month old, and I thought it was so unfair that I barely even got to experience being her mother. There wasn't anything I could do for her. I couldn't feed her or change her; I couldn't even speak to her. I guess I just figured she would be happier being held by someone that could give her the attention she deserved.

My mom would hold Casey above me so that she could see me, and I realized just how smart she was when, one day, she did the most amazing thing. She had watched and heard me "cluck" to communicate so many times, and this one time, as she looked at me and my head was turned, she clucked to get my attention. I was so proud of her and excited that I finally had a way of communicating with her as well.

On March 9, Day 16, CBC and Global, two local news companies, came in to do a story on me. One of my girlfriends had thought that the media would be interested in hearing my story, so she reached out to them. They were interested because many people had never even heard of Guillain-Barré syndrome, and it would promote great public awareness about the illness. They knew that our story would reach people not only because the illness is so devastating, but also because of the added fact that I had just given birth to a baby a few weeks earlier.

My mom did up my makeup for the interview, and although I don't actually recall doing the interview, we watched it on the news later that evening and the following day. I was famous! I must have thought I was a bigger deal than I really was because I kept telling my girlfriend to call Oprah. I was actually convinced she would come to Canada and do a story on me too! My friends laughed and told me that Oprah was on her final season and had already picked all her last shows so she wouldn't be able to do a story on me. I was quite disappointed.

By mid March, my paralysis was at its worst. It had spread upward to my face, and I could no longer move my mouth or even smile. All I could do was blink, and even then I couldn't keep my eyes looking straight. These were one of my darkest times, and I quickly lost hope again. I struggled enough as it was to talk with my family without the use of my voice or my hands, and now that all that I could do was blink, how was anyone going to understand me? James told me this was the hardest time for him because he didn't know how I would be able to communicate anymore.

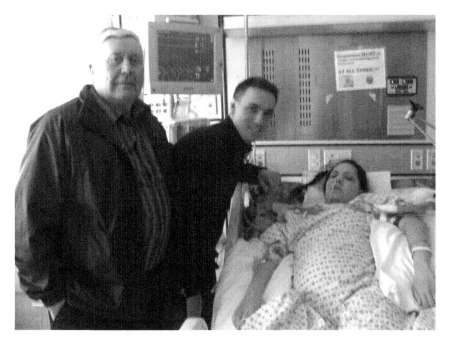

My cousin, grandpa and me

The ICU staff wanted to cheer us up, and they suggested we do a date night. They would wheel in a big screen TV with a DVD player for us so that we could have a movie night. And even though I was completely paralysed and could barely communicate in words, I spelled out to my cousin to bring in Beef Jerky and Skittles for James for our date, two of his favourite snacks.

That night was one of our favourite nights. James was amazed that I had thought of his favourite snacks even in my condition. My paralysis had even improved slightly that day, and my smile started to improve.

We watched *Due Date*, which was hilarious, and when I laughed, I had a half-smile that made James laugh. My nausea was also gone for the entire movie so I actually felt good for a change. Every Saturday night thereafter became movie date night, when my mom would go home and James and Casey would stay overnight with me.

On March 13, *Day 19*, my family saw a tiny movement in my fingers. It was the first time I had moved them in over two weeks. This meant that I was improving. I had finally hit my plateau!

I was finally getting stronger. I was able to slightly move my arms and shoulders a little bit throughout that week. My family was ecstatic, and they made a star for the milestone and put it above my bed. Although I had every reason to be happy, I wasn't. I was still in pain, I was still nauseated, and I still didn't have my life back. I really didn't care that I was starting to move again.

The following day, the doctors wanted to start getting me up in the chair. My mom was leery. I was barely moving my fingers, and she did not think I was ready to be hoisted up in the air by a lift yet. They assured her that it would be fine.

They rolled me over, which made me cry in pain, and placed the sling under my body. The sling was then attached to the lift, and they started lifting me up in the air. I immediately started bawling because it hurt so unbelievably bad, everywhere. I couldn't hold my head up, so it hurt my neck. I was practically being bent in half, so it hurt my back, and my legs had that excruciating pain shooting through them. The nurses and my family quickly figured out a way to hold my head and legs so it wasn't as bad, but it involved six people helping out.

I was placed into a chair that reclined all the way back. I was so hot from being moved around that I started to have a major hot flash, and my family had to soak my face with wet cloths. After I cooled down, they put Casey on my lap and rolled me out of my hospital room. What an ordeal- just to get out of bed.

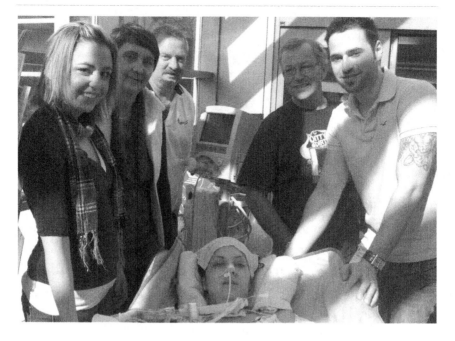

My first time up in the chair—with my best friend, my parents and James

It was *Day 20*, and it was fantastic to finally see outside my room. My whole family was there that day, and along with a nurse and an RT, who wheeled the ventilator beside me, we all went down to the lobby. I felt like a spectacle. So many people were looking at us, and I'm sure I looked like I was dying.

I was so hot from being moved around that we decided to go outside. The fresh air felt so nice that I finally felt like I wasn't in a sauna. It was sunny outside, but probably only zero degrees, so everyone was cold, but I couldn't have been happier. I was in just my hospital gown and felt it was the perfect temperature. People would walk by me and stare; they must have thought my family was so cruel that they were not even covering me up.

The doctors wanted me to try and stay up in the chair as long as I could since the movement was so good for my lungs, but after only an hour, my back was aching so badly that I wanted to get back to bed. The lift back was almost as painful and just as terrifying, and I was absolutely relieved when I was finally in my bed. I never thought I would actually be happy to be back in my room, but it was where I felt the most comfortable.

My immune system was weak, so I was more susceptible to catching a hospital infection than the average person. I was constantly having my urinary catheter changed, which put me at a higher risk to contracting an ESBL bladder infection, and it wasn't long before I tested positive for one. I had no symptoms of the infection, which meant I was just a carrier, therefore, there was no reason to treat it. The bacteria would eventually work itself through my body, but until it did, we would need to take precautions to ensure that I didn't pass on the bacteria to another patient.

Anyone entering my room would now need to wear a yellow gown and gloves. This included nurses and doctors, which made things a lot more time-consuming. Every time they left to get something, they would have to disrobe, take off their gloves, wash their hands and get what they needed, and then put on a gown and gloves again. We weren't sure how to protect Casey as she wouldn't fit into a gown, so for a few days they had us place her in a pillowcase. It didn't work very well, so it didn't last long, and everyone agreed to keep their hands clean whenever holding her.

I couldn't seem to catch a break as shortly after, I also contracted fungal bacteria in my mouth, called thrush, from all the antibiotics I was on. The bacteria made my mouth extremely pasty and covered my tongue in a thick white paste. I was put on another medication that I would swish around in my mouth and spit out. It took about a month to get rid of the thrush, but with the ESBL infection I wasn't as lucky. I had it the entire time I was in the hospital, and it didn't go away until well after I was home.

Almost every day, they had me use the speaking valve, and each time I used it, I got better and better at it. On St. Patrick's Day, *Day*

24, I was able to say Happy St. Patty's Day to Casey, and another time, when James was at home, I was able to speak to him over the phone.

They tried to get me into the chair everyday, to improve the condition of my lungs and also to lift my spirits by getting me out of my room. But I absolutely hated it. Being lifted into the chair was always painful; sitting in the chair was always uncomfortable; and being outside always felt strange to me. As soon as I thought I had been outside long enough to make them happy, I would ask to go back to my room.

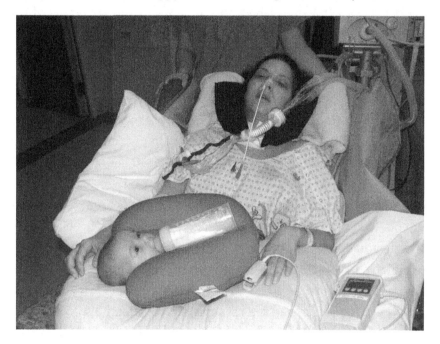

Chair rides with Casey

But the plus side to the chair was that I was finally able to have my hair washed. I had been lying in bed for weeks, and it felt fantastic to finally have this done. The nurses leaned me back as far as I could go in the chair and poured water over my head into a basin. It felt amazing. My hair was getting so long that it took a really long time, so it was only something the nurses could do once a week.

It was March 18, *Day 25*, when they decided to remove the NG feeding tube that went through my nose. I had been in the hospital for a little over three weeks, and this tube was generally only used in the short term. It would be a lot more comfortable for me to insert a feeding tube right into my stomach.

I was put out by means of anesthesia for the procedure, and they inserted the feeding tube through a small incision they made about two inches above and to the left of my belly button.

When I woke up, I was much more comfortable; I no longer had this tube in my nose and down my throat, and I couldn't even feel the tube in my stomach. But the only downfall was that now when they would feed me through the tube, and when they would crush up pills to put into the tube, I could literally feel everything entering my stomach. The thought of it made me feel sick, and I felt even more nauseated than before. I just wanted to throw up, but I couldn't; all I could do was dry heave. It broke my family's hearts to watch me heave over and over all day long.

Exactly a week after my fingers had first moved, on March 19, the nightmare started all over again. Seeing that November 19 is my birthday and June 19 is James' birthday, and that we started dating and were married on the 19th, we had hoped that this would be a good day. However, it was the complete opposite. The paralysis returned, and I could no longer move anything, including my face, for the second time. For days, I lay completely still with my family waiting for any kind of movement, but nothing happened. No matter how hard I tried, I couldn't move a thing.

The doctors told my family I must have not hit my plateau yet. So until I reached that point, I would not start improving. We were all devastated.

My friends came up with the most amazing idea ever. They came in to tell me what they had planned. They were going to throw a fundraiser for James, Casey, and me to raise money for us. They knew that even once I was out of the hospital, it would be a long time before I would be able to work again, so they wanted to make things financially easier for us.

Their plan was to get as many things as they could donated, and they would have a silent auction for people to bid on the items. They started making plans for it, made the announcement on Facebook, and immediately people started messaging them with things to donate for the fundraiser.

Every day, someone would tell me of ten more people that had donated something. Our friends were overwhelmed by the amount of support pouring in; people were donating anything and everything; hockey tickets, autographed jerseys, salon gift cards, photography gift cards, restaurant gift cards, bath sets, golf bags, guitars, pictures, concert tickets, gift baskets, shoes, and quilts, to name just a few items.

Some people wanted to donate money directly to us instead, so checks starting pouring in for our family as well. The money came in so handy. On top of our expenses at home, we now had expenses here as well. Between all the food and snacks my family needed while here, we also had to pay for parking every day, which was extremely expensive.

People also started donating things to us directly. Some people donated gift cards for grocery stores. James was now able to buy food and snacks to bring into the hospital, and he didn't have to worry about the added expense of that every week. Another great donation was diapers. Boxes came in by the dozens, and we were so relieved to not have to worry about that expense either. But the most amazing of them all was from Enfamil. James' auntie had called the formula company and told them of our story, and they donated over sixty tins of formula to us.

CTV news also contacted us to do another news story on us, and my girlfriend made the announcement about the Fundraiser and how to donate on the CTV News.

The fundraiser was on the night of March 26, *Day 33*, and my mom stayed with me while all my friends and family went out to support me.

They set up a laptop with Skype so they were able to send a shout-out to me live, with me on my mom's laptop watching at the hospital. I was pretty out of it so I didn't quite realize the extent of it all, but the next day my friends came and told me that there were over four hundred people in attendance and that they had raised over thirty thousand dollars for us. It was such a huge relief to know that, on top of everything we were dealing with, we wouldn't need to worry about money.

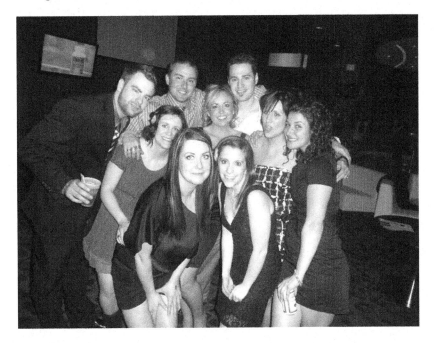

My friends and family at the fundraiser

By the end of March, I was even more aware of what was going on around me. I was in a lot less pain, so I was on a lot less medication. Although the skin on my legs was still very sensitive, the rest of my body wasn't as bad, and the pain in my back was a lot better.

The past five weeks in intensive care had been a blur; I don't remember a large portion of it, and the days had flown by. I was still completely paralyzed and unable to move an inch from the neck down and still waiting to hit my plateau.

Althought I felt more aware, my memory was still not quite there yet. One day, when my girlfriend, who had always had a BlackBerry, came in with her brand-new iPhone, I made a comment about it. She told me that I had seen it several times now and that every single time I saw it, I had said something. I had no recollection of this.

To make matter worse, my eyes become affected, and almost overnight, I started seeing double. It made me dizzy, and it made things way worse with my nausea. I had felt sick but hadn't been able to throw up. I now went from being nauseous some of the time to nauseous and throwing up all day long. I would cry and cry as I violently threw up over and over again.

The nurses suggested that I cover one eye at a time by wearing an eyepatch. It was a simple black fabric patch that the nurses taped to my face over my eye. It definitely helped with the double vision, so I wore it anytime I was awake. We switched eyes every other day to make sure one eye didn't become stronger than the other, but whenever we changed eyes and had the patch off, I would get dizzy and immediately start throwing up.

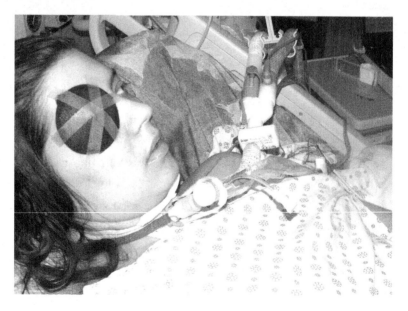

Eyepatch

On the positive side of things, my family and friends were becoming pros at reading my lips, so I no longer used the communication board at all. I was also able to make a very faint sound with my lips, so it almost sounded like I was whispering. It made things so much easier, and we were pretty much able to communicate completely. I was also becoming a pro on the speaking valve and was doing trials up to half an hour a day. It was fantastic to be able to have that time to actually speak with my family and friends every day.

Also, the doctors thought my bladder was ready to start working on its own, so they removed the urinary catheter in hopes that I could start urinating again. They hoped that I would be able to feel the urge to pee so that I could start asking for a bedpan when I needed one.

The first time I felt like I had to pee, I was so relieved; it meant that I wasn't paralyzed down there. But when it came down to it, I just couldn't do it. I tried and tried, but nothing came out. The nurses tried to help by running water for me, but it didn't work; I just couldn't go on my own. I didn't have the strength in my bladder to let it go.

They weren't ready to give up and put the catheter back in, but they would need to get the urine out of my bladder somehow, so they decided to do a straight catheter, also known as an in-and-out catheter. It was basically the same as the catheter I had before, only this time the catheter tube would be inserted only to drain the bladder, and as soon as it was done, it would be removed.

The procedure was done with two nurses, and as soon as it started, I wished I could have tried longer to go on my own. I had gone through so much pain in the last five weeks, but this was the worst. It seemed to take forever as they tried to put the tube up my urethra. It felt like they were taking razor blades to my crotch. I cried and screamed for it to just be over, with James holding my hand. Finally, once the catheter was in the right position, my bladder started to drain. The pain lessened, and I was so thankful it was over.

The next time I had to pee, I tried for a lot longer to go, and after a good solid twenty minutes or so of trying, and with the help of running water, I finally went. I was so unbelievably relieved; I never thought going pee could make me so happy. As long as I didn't have to go through an in-and-out catheter again though, I would be happy.

But that was not the last time. Regrettably, I had to be straight catheterized many more times. Sometimes I had no problem urinating on my own, but at other times I just couldn't go, even when I felt like I had to so badly. Finally, after a few days of torture, they decided to put the more permanent catheter back in. I had it in for about a week and then we tried things again.

This time, my bladder was back on track, and I had no more issues with it. Whenever I needed to pee, I was supposed to let the nurse know, and they would put a bedpan under me to use. However, I quickly learned that I did not have control over my bodily functions. I could feel it after it happened, but most of the time, I could not feel anything leading up to it, and I had no control. Sometimes I used the bedpan, but most of the time, the nurses diapered me or "put me in a brief," and I was changed just like a baby.

Whenever the nurses would clean and change me, I felt sick to my stomach and would constantly mouth the words "I'm sorry" to them. I had barely gotten used to doing this for my own daughter, let alone having someone I barely knew do this for me. I was disgusted and embarrassed that they had to do this, and I was completely humiliated. I would, however, take this over a straight catheter any day.

I was getting up in the chair every day now, for at least an hour, and when it was nice out, we sat outside, and when it was not, we sat in the cafeteria lounge.

James planned to bring our dogs in one day to visit me when I was outside, and I was so excited to see them. James called our room that morning, *Day 36*, and informed me that the dogs had gotten out of our yard and taken off. I guess I told him to not even think about coming into the hospital until he had found them, although I don't remember saying that.

About an hour and a half later, one of our dogs, Bentley, showed up at the front door of our house. But our other dog, Hugo, was still missing. James and some of our friends searched the entire neighborhood all afternoon but couldn't find him anywhere. James starting panicking and posted Hugo's picture and our phone number on a local Lost Dog website in the hope that someone would find him.

About six hours later, he received a call from the Humane Society asking if he had lost his dog. Someone had brought in a dog to them that had been hit by a car, and they had checked the website. James rushed over right away, and luckily Hugo was OK. He had a few scrapes and bruises and a little bit of road rash, but he was more shaken up than anything.

The following day, James brought them to the hospital to see me. The whole time I had been in the hospital, it had been very cold and snowy, but this day was the nicest spring day we had had yet, being plus eight degrees and very sunny.

James parked the car and walked over with our dogs, and they were so excited to see me. They ran over as fast as they could and seemed so happy to finally see me again. Bentley tried to jump on me and my family held him back so he wouldn't hurt me, but Hugo seemed almost upset, like he was hurt that I had left him for so long. He was still pretty jittery from the car accident so I assume that was a part of it too.

The nurses were happy to hear that James had brought the dogs in to see me as they knew that it would put me in a good mood. One nurse had really noticed my mood lately and told me that in the beginning she'd seen me have both good and bad days, but it seemed like I never had any good days anymore. She asked me to remember when I had had my last good day, and I told her I didn't remember ever having any good days in the hospital.

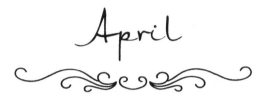

April

Casey got pinkeye at the beginning of April, and for the first time, I didn't get to see my baby for four days. James stayed home with her, and I missed them both so much. However, my brother was back from out of town work, and it was always nice to have him visit. Every time he saw me, he couldn't believe how much better I looked since the last time. I wasn't on as much medication so I was much more awake than before.

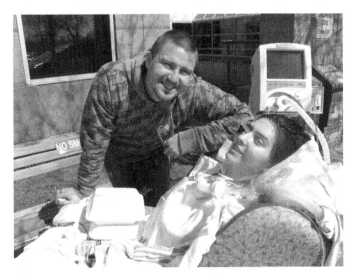

My brother and me outside

Although it would still be a while yet, the plan was for me to eventually come off the ventilator and be moved out of the ICU into another ward. The RTs started doing negative inspiratory force (NIF) tests to measure my lung strength. NIF tests were one of the several indicators used to tell them when I was ready to start being weaned off the ventilator.

Basically, I had to breathe into a device that measured the strength of my breath. The first time I did it, I could not believe how hard it was. I struggled to catch my breath, and I was so hot immediately afterward that I thought I was going to faint. I was panicking. My family patted my face with a cold cloth and helped cool me down. After a few minutes, I caught my breath and was able to relax.

The NIF level should be around negative thirty cm H_2O; a normal person can have an NIF level around negative forty-five cm H_2O, and the first time I did it, I was only at negative five cm H_2O. They did NIF tests every few days, and for the longest time, I remained at negative five cm H_2O. Every time almost made me faint, and I absolutely dreaded when the RTs came in to do them.

We prepared for them by getting cold cloths ready, and they then patted my face to cool me down. I couldn't believe how much work it took just to breathe in. Some days, when I was more tired or nauseated than usual, I would ask for them to come back and do the test at a later time.

When it had been quite a while between tests, the RT asked me if I would do one for him. I said no, that I just wasn't up to it that day again. But he really wanted to see where I was, and insisted. I was frustrated and felt anxious. I had my mom get the cold cloth ready, and I breathed in as hard as I could. Then I had her pat my forehead to cool me down. I was still the same as the last time I had done it. I was so exhausted and instantly felt more nauseated than before.

My respiratory therapist was proud of me; he knew that I really didn't want to do the test, and he knew that it made me feel sick. As he walked out of the room, he turned back and told me that because I did the NIF test for him, he would let me stay at his vacation home in Phoenix once I got out of the hospital. I had the biggest smile on my face. I whispered "Seriously, after all this, I'm definitely going to need a vacation."

I was still completely paralysed and very depressed, but some things were actually improving. I could handle being up in the chair for longer periods of time, and I wasn't as hot all the time anymore either. I rarely wore a blanket and almost always had my gown pulled up as high as it could possibly go, but I no longer needed a cloth on my head all the time. My pain and sensitivity seemed to be gradually decreasing as well, and on *Day 43*, I even went an entire day without needing any "top-ups" of medication.

I didn't require as much suctioning of my trach, which was great, because coughing and gagging a hundred times a day was really hard on me. My mood seemed to be getting a little better, and once on my speaking valve, instead of talking, I sang along to the song "Bubbly," by Colbie Caillet, on my iPod. James smiled and laughed and videotaped me singing. He was a lot happier these days too as many things were definitely improving with me, and I'm sure it was nice to finally see me in a better mood.

But things quickly came crashing down on April 7, *Day 45*. Although certain things with me were improving, I still hadn't hit my plateau. Most GBS patients hit their plateau after two to three weeks. It had been almost six weeks, and I still hadn't hit it yet. The doctors were beginning to think that my overall recovery would take a lot longer than they had hoped.

They told my mom that morning that they thought I would be in the hospital for at least a year. My mom was devastated and struggled to find a way to tell James when he got to the hospital that morning.

When James arrived, he had worse news than we could even imagine. One of our friends with whom James had been friends since Junior High had committed suicide. What made the news even more devastating was that he was supposed to be coming in that very day to visit me.

I don't even know how James kept it together. He was dealing with his wife being in the hospital, being a full-time dad to Casey, and now one of his friends had died. My mom decided not to tell James what the doctors had said about my recovery as she just didn't think he could handle any more bad news right now.

April 9, *Day 47*, was definitely one of the hardest days I had had in the hospital. I was feeling the most nauseated I'd ever been and spent the entire day vomiting. It was the sickest I had ever felt in my entire life. One of the nurses even thought that maybe I had a stomach bug because I was way sicker than usual. I begged her to do something, and she tried different types of medications, but nothing worked. I cried to my family, actually believing there was something they could do, but there was nothing they could do to make me feel better.

I was throwing up nonstop for over an hour when my nurse finally decided to try something different. She wanted to drain the contents of my stomach, in the hope that maybe I had something in there that was making me sick. She would need to put the NG tube back into my stomach through my nose and pump my stomach through the tube.

I was terrified of going through any more pain, and I asked her if it was going to hurt. All she said was that it was going to be very uncomfortable, but that she needed me to just keep swallowing. She went and got the tube, and before I even had a chance to take a breath and prepare for it, she stuck the tube as hard and as far up into my nose as she could.

It wasn't particularly painful, but it was definitely extremely uncomfortable. I could feel the tube coming down into the back of my throat, and she told me to just keep swallowing, which brought the tube down into my stomach. My stomach was drained into a container beside my bed, and after a few hours, it still hadn't helped. I had nothing left to throw up, so instead, I dry heaved.

I hated the feeling of the tube in my throat, and it was very uncomfortable every time I swallowed. The nurse gave me a spray that numbed my throat so I wouldn't feel the tube. But after she sprayed my throat, not only could I not feel the tube anymore, but also my throat was now numb, and it felt like I couldn't breathe properly. I started having a panic attack. I felt like I couldn't breathe, and I thought I was going to die.

The nurses gave me a medication to help me relax, and after a few minutes I calmed down. The throat spray eventually wore off, and I was able to breathe comfortably again. My stomach was finally emptied as well, but unfortunately, it hadn't helped at all with my nausea. I was still as sick as I ever was.

Later that evening, out of nowhere, I moved my fingers. My family was completely shocked to see movement after the day I had and after all this time. It had been three weeks since I had last moved anything on my body and five weeks overall of being paralyzed. James and my mom were excited; this could mean that I had actually reached my plateau this time and that my paralysis would start fading. They made a star above my bed and immediately made phone calls and announced on Facebook that I was finally moving again.

They were so unbelievably happy, but it was hard for them because when they looked at me, I looked so depressed. I was so extremely nauseous that I couldn't be happy about my hands moving. My mom kept telling me that it meant that I was getting better, but I didn't listen. In my eyes, I was not getting better. I felt worse than I had ever felt.

That night, with a new nurse on shift, I continued vomiting all night long. She would give me meds for my nausea whenever she could, but I was only able to have them every certain number of hours.

After throwing up continuously for hours and hours, I begged the nurse to do something. She said there was nothing she could do for me and that I needed to "grin and bear it."

I was fuming. I could not "grin and bear it." I could not do this any longer. That was it. I was throwing in the towel. I was ready to give up.

I couldn't handle this life anymore, so I told my mom that I wanted to die.

She said that she was not going to let me die now that I was just finally starting to get better. I didn't care. I just knew that I was done and that I was ready to die. I begged her to do something about it; I knew there was nothing I could do since I was paralyzed. My mom just kept telling me I needed to hold on for Casey's sake. I would eventually get better.

I knew my mom wasn't going to let me die. So I impatiently waited until I could be given more meds for my nausea.

The next time the nurse came in, I saw that it was a different nurse as mine was busy with something else. I asked her if there was anything she could do for me, and she said she would at least ask the doctor if I could be given something early. It took what felt like forever, as the doctor was busy, but eventually I was given some more medication. By this time, it was almost morning, and either I was so exhausted or the meds helped because I eventually fell asleep.

The next morning, I didn't feel any better. I hadn't even been awake for ten minutes, and I was already throwing up again. I was exhausted. I was not going to do this anymore. I didn't have the strength in me to fight anymore. I immediately asked my mom to get me one of the respiratory therapists. I had no control over things, but I knew they did. My mom knew exactly what I was going to say to the RT, and she told her what to expect when she came to talk to me.

When the RT came in, I told her I needed her help. First, I asked her for a DNR. When I was first admitted to the ICU, I had signed a form stating that if I were to stop breathing, they would perform CPR on me right away. A DNR, or a Do Not Resuscitate, is an order that in the event I stopped breathing, they would respect my wishes and I would not undergo CPR; I would be let go naturally. I wanted her to change my form to a DNR. I couldn't go on living like this anymore, and I wanted her to take me off the respirator. I was bawling and begged her to just disconnect me so I could die. I could see her fighting back tears, and she told me that I couldn't give up. I had come so far, and I had a baby girl that needed me. I realized she wasn't going to help me either. Although I was so ready to give up, I knew I had no choice but to keep on fighting. We made a star for my fingers moving and put it up above my bed. I made it through yet another horrific day.

Our friend's funeral was early the following week, and it was devastating to me that I was unable to go and say good-bye to our friend. I wanted so badly to be there for my husband. It broke my heart that I couldn't be there the way he had been there for me these past few months. Everyone was asking James how I was doing, and he was happy to let everyone know that I was slowly getting better, at least physically.

That week, I continued to move my fingers a little bit more each day. But the nausea was still there every single day, so I really didn't care that I was moving. I was, however, on the least amount of medication for pain yet. I finally felt like I was back in reality, instead of constantly being high as a kite and not knowing what was going on around me.

The past few months had flown by, partly because of all the meds but also because I had probably slept half of the time. But now, I was finally awake all day long and was fully aware what day it was. And time really started to slow down. I remember many, many days where I simply stared at the clock, watching the hands move all day long. I remember looking up and then, what seemed like hours later, looking up again to see that only twenty minutes had gone by, and tears would just flow down my face.

We got into a pretty good daily routine, and every day started to feel the same as the one before. Every morning I would wake up, and I would watch the morning news. I felt very isolated in my hospital room, and it felt good to see what was going on in the rest of the world. My mom would start my day by brushing my teeth, and she would use the suction to remove the toothpaste from my mouth, since I wasn't allowed to swallow anything.

My respiratory therapist would then come in to suction my trach, which sometimes made me puke, sometimes not. Every time, it always made me cough fiercely for a few minutes. I still loved it when the RTs came in, though; they always seemed interested in me as a person and not just a patient. They always talked to me about how things were going and really treated me like their friend.

I wanted to know right away who my nurse was for the day, and my mom would go and find out for me. Anytime that she came back and told me I had a nurse that I had never had yet, I would start feeling anxious. I was absolutely terrified of having new nurses.

The nurses were trained to bend the knee when turning patients, but this caused me excruciating pain so I was log rolled instead. The nurses that had never worked with me before wouldn't know this and would always try to bend my leg, leaving me in tears.

I was also so hypersensitive that I hated being touched, and the ones that knew that were extra gentle with me. Those that didn't know constantly hurt me with what seemed like harsh movements.

I also wasn't sure how they would deal with me throwing up all day long. Some of the nurses were more caring about it, holding my hair back as I puked or rubbing my forehead, while others seemed to care less about it. They figured they had done all they could do, and they simply went about their tasks as I threw up for hours.

The ones that were assigned to me more often would talk a little about their personal lives to us. They would tell us stories of their kids, their vacations, what their husbands did for a living, etc. It was so nice to have a conversation with people, and I truly felt like they cared about me as a friend. I definitely had my favorites, and it always put me at ease if I ended up with a nurse that I had had before.

Once my nurse came in and checked my vitals, she would go get all my medications ready. My mom would then do my range of motion exercises, and she was happy that I was actually starting to slightly push back with my hands and arms.

When my nurse came back, she would give me my pain medications and then prepare for my sponge bath. This was definitely one of the favorite parts of my day. First of all, the pain medication gave me an instant high and instant pain relief. Secondly, the bath was fantastic. The nurses used my own body wash that James had brought in for me, which was Aveeno Body Wash for babies. It always reminded me of when I had bathed Casey during those first few weeks at home.

I was wiped down with warm soapy water from head to toe, and it was nice to feel cleaner every morning, especially since I only had my hair washed about once a week in a basin. Bath time was also the only time I was completely comfortable temperature wise. I was still overly warm all the time, and my body finally felt cool from the water against my skin. I actually started asking for warm blankets to cover up in. But after only a few minutes in the blanket, I would start to overheat again very quickly.

My nurse would then give me the rest of my pills for the morning by first crushing them and adding water and then injecting them with a syringe into my feeding tube in my stomach. I hated this part of the day; it still made me feel sick when the fluid splashed around in my belly. It was almost clockwork for me to start feeling nauseated within five to ten minutes of getting my meds. I think my stomach just couldn't handle it, and once I was nauseous, I was sick for most of the day.

My family and I could not believe how much medication I was still being given. Aside from the pain meds, I was also on several different meds to keep my bowels moving and to try and help with my nausea, a blood thinner to prevent blood clots, and two different antidepressants, which not only helped with my mood but also with the nerve pain that caused sensitivity in my skin. I was also on a few others that I simply don't remember.

I was given tube feed, a type of nutritional liquid, as my main source of food. This was also given to me through my feeding tube, and this as well made me feel sick to my stomach. At one time, when things were really bad with my nausea, I refused the tube feed in the hope that I would feel better without it. I felt like I was being given way too many medications and this one time I just wanted it all to stop. However, I was quickly advised not to refuse it as I really needed the nutrients, even though I never ever felt hungry.

Some days, my mom would read me my Facebook posts and messages. It was always uplifting to hear all the comforting words people sent.

James and Casey would come in around eleven o'clock every morning, so he had time to get things done around the house. I was so proud of him for taking on the duties I had at home, as well as taking care of Casey. He was doing such a wonderful job, being an amazing husband and father, and a part of me wondered how on earth he was keeping it together. I constantly had nurses commenting on how amazing a husband I had and how he had really stepped up to the plate. James didn't really get what he was doing that was so amazing. He felt that he was just doing what any husband would do for their family in this time of need.

Once James and Casey were in, I would get up in the chair. It was such a huge ordeal getting me up in the chair, but we had done it so many times now that James and my mom were now pros. They did it so well that I would only get up in the chair if both of them were there to help with the move.

First, we would put on my foot splints, which my mom called Moon Boots, as that's what they looked like, and then they would roll me to place the sling underneath my body. This was so painful. Then James held my legs so they didn't dangle. As they lifted me in the air, a nurse held my head, and my mom helped my torso move up and across my bed and into the chair. The transfer was still making me so hot that one time I even fainted after not being able to catch my breath.

Once I cooled down, we would go downstairs to the lobby and sit outside or in the lounge. An RT always came with us to wheel my ventilator along beside me. My nurse came too, and the ones that knew me well were always prepared for the trip by bringing a kidney basin for me to throw up in case I got sick and a cold cloth to wipe down my face in case I overheated.

In the lobby, we would pass the kiosks selling different things such as shoes and purses, and those being two of my favourite things to shop for; my family would always point them out to me as I wheeled by. I, however, had no interest in them. I was paralyzed and lived in a hospital; I had no use for purses and shoes. Day after day, my family would stop to see the different things they were selling, and I always waited impatiently as they looked. I didn't understand why they thought I would want to look at things that I couldn't use or wear. It only reminded me of how terrible my life had become.

After my trip in the chair, I would get my afternoon meds and then we would do more range of motion exercises. I spent my afternoons sleeping, watching TV, and hanging out with James and Casey, James' parents, my parents, my brothers, or anyone else that had stopped by to visit for the day. I still had the odd friend visiting in the evenings but there were definitely not as many as before. I loved it when people came to visit, but I hated having to throw up in front of them and didn't want them to see me cry.

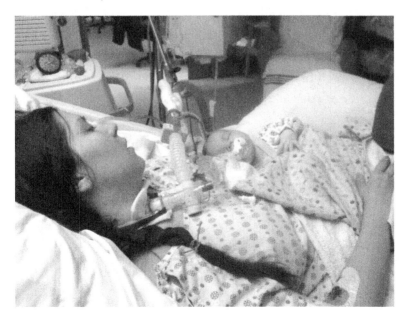

Napping with Casey

At night, after James and Casey left, my mom and I would do one last round of range of motion exercises. I would get my evening meds, my mom would brush my teeth, and we would go to bed. My mom always made sure the lights were out by ten o'clock, just in case I ended up throwing up in the middle of the night and didn't get very much sleep. In the first few weeks, I had slept whenever I was tired, and now I was finally on a good routine. I was given a sleeping pill so I was able to fall asleep fairly quickly, and the doctor even put in a Do Not Disturb order so that I would not be disturbed through the night. I was finally at a place where I could find a comfortable way to sleep; I needed a specific pillow for my neck, a pillow in between my legs, and the blanket that one of my girlfriends had made for me.

Although I had no trouble falling asleep because of the pill, there were many nights I would wake up sick and spend an hour or so throwing up. The nurses always came with a top-up, but the best nurses would spend a few minutes comforting me and rubbing my forehead, telling me that I would get through this. Sometimes they would change me, which was a huge ordeal. It felt very invasive being sprawled on my bed with lights shining down on me while they cleaned me up. I had no choice but to just lie there and cry. The best nights were definitely when I would sleep all through the night. And when the morning came, we would start each day all over again.

My family would say that the beginning weeks were the hardest for them as they were unfamiliar with my illness and didn't know what to expect. They had waited weeks for me to show any signs of improvement, so now that I was actually improving every day, they were a lot happier.

But for me, this was the hardest time. I could handle the pain; I could not handle being sick twenty-four hours a day. I was severely depressed. I didn't care about my life at all anymore. My mom would offer to do my makeup, and my friends would offer to pluck my eyebrows, but I would always decline; I no longer cared what I looked like. I just didn't see the point when I would rather be dead.

The meds for my nausea didn't ever seem to help anymore, and after hours and hours of throwing up, I would cry to my family and ask when I was going to get better. I just wanted my life to go back to the way it was. My mom kept telling me that I already was getting better, that I had improved so much since the beginning, but I didn't understand. To me, I was just as bad as I ever was. I felt like I was in a nightmare that I just couldn't wake up from. I had a pit in my stomach that never went away.

I suffered from panic attacks quite often as many times I worried that I wasn't able to breathe. Being on the ventilator was extremely hard on me. Struggling with every single breath I took was very difficult and made me feel very claustrophobic.

I also struggled with everything that was going on. Several times a day, I would lie in my bed and think about everything that had happened to me. I would think about how I could barely move my own body, how I couldn't even enjoy my little girl, how I lived in a hospital, and it was just too much. My heart raced, my breathing accelerated, and I would start to have another panic attack. I just wanted to scream as loud as I could and throw my arms and legs up in the air, but I couldn't. No sounds came out, and nothing moved. Instead, I would arch my back and violently shake my head back and forth, with tears streaming down my face.

Once I had such a severe panic attack that I felt like the walls were closing in around me, and I told my mom to take down all the photos around the room. She didn't understand why, but to me, everything was just too much. There was too much going on around me, and I wanted everything taken off the walls. My mom worried that once I felt better, I would want it all back up, so she asked if it was OK if she just took down the pink boas, which I agreed to. Whenever I had panic attacks, I was always given a medication to help me relax. I wouldn't necessarily say that it worked, but it definitely helped to take the edge off.

The panic attacks were getting so bad that my mom even called in a hypnotherapist, in the hope that he could help me relax when I felt anxious. He told me to try and get into a deep meditative state, and whenever I felt anxious or in pain, to focus on a specific color that made me happy. I could also focus on a specific time in my life, like my wedding day or lying on a beach. It was very difficult to try and focus on anything but my troubled breathing, but I did my best.

I also had my mom call the man that had GBS before, hoping that maybe he could give me some advice on how to deal with things. I felt I was not able to emotionally deal with things at all, and maybe he would be able to lift my spirits again, like he had before.

He and his wife came in and brought me a poster that read, "Courage does not always roar. It's also the soft voice, at day's end, I'll try again tomorrow." I felt like he was the only one that understood what I was going through. People kept telling me how strong I was, and how proud of me they were, and I just couldn't understand why. I didn't think I was dealing with things well at all. Little did they know that I was hoping that I would just die. But that poster reminded me that I didn't need to be handling things well to be strong. I just needed to get through each day one minute at a time.

He brought up that now that I was moving my hands and arms, things would probably start progressing quickly, as they had with him. Every day, he was able to move something new. I was very excited and hoped that the same thing would happen to me. I also asked him if he was as sick as I was and how he dealt with it, and he said he was very sick as well, and that one day it just went away on its own. He said most medications didn't work for him, although one medication had helped, but the side effects were too harsh. The medication was a synthetic version of THC, the main substance found in marijuana, and although it did take away his nausea, he didn't like how stoned it made him, so he asked to come off it.

I was desperate and willing to try anything, so I had my mom take down the name of the drug, and the next time I felt I needed it, I would ask my doctor to try it.

The time had finally come, to start the weaning process from the ventilator. The RTs set my ventilator to a spontaneous mode of ventilation called Pressure Support. Essentially, instead of the ventilator mechanically making me breathe, I was now initiating my own breaths, which would then trigger the ventilator to deliver support. It was a lot more work for me to breathe, and I constantly felt short of breath when I was on it. At first, the RTs would let me know when they had switched me over to Pressure Support, but because I knew, I was more aware of how hard it was to take in a breath. I would only last a few hours on it in the beginning because I would always start to have a panic attack; I felt like I couldn't breathe. I was given more medication for the panic attacks, but the only thing that really helped was to just take me off Pressure Support. I eventually realized that a lot of it was in my mind, so I asked the RTs not to tell me when they would switch me over. Without knowing, I didn't focus on my breathing, and eventually I was able to last almost twelve straight hours on it.

The next step after the Pressure Support was for me to try breathing on my own. April 15, *Day 53*, was the first time I would be breathing without the ventilator. To take me off, they used a different type of speaking valve that allowed me to breathe completely on my own, as well as talk with my friends and family. Breathing was extremely difficult, and I was terrified I was going to die from lack of oxygen, so I only lasted three minutes. But everyone was thrilled. Even three minutes was something to be very proud of. And of course, we made a star and put it above my bed.

That weekend was the first time in a very long time that I wasn't sick all day. My nurse seized the moment and decided to spend some of her shift making my day even more enjoyable. She pulled out my makeup bag and did my makeup for me, brushed out my hair, and shaved my legs. She even put on my headband that looked like the one she had on, and the nurses all loved that she spent the day making me beautiful and said we even looked like twins. That was definitely one of my best days.

When I was able to move my shoulders and my neck for the first time that afternoon, I was actually excited about my movement, but only because I wasn't nauseated for once. My family was thrilled that I could be a part of their happiness and to finally see me excited over something. I also did my second time on the speaking valve off the ventilator and this time, I lasted ten minutes. My mom was overjoyed to finally see me smile for the first time in weeks.

My nausea-free weekend was short-lived, and late Sunday afternoon I started vomiting and couldn't stop. I cried and cried and then I thought about the THC drug and had my mom get the doctor. When I asked him about it, he told me one of the doctors had actually given it to me at the beginning the first time I ever felt sick. But when the next doctor came on shift the following week, he felt it wasn't working and had stopped it. We told him just how frustrating this was for us as every week a new doctor would have a new idea on how to treat me. But when their week was done, and the next doctor came on, they would have a different idea and would start me on something completely different. The doctor agreed that the unit needed to work together and communicate better amongst each other and said that he would talk to them about it. As for my nausea, he was certainly willing to try this drug again. I asked him if I would feel too high, and he said it was possible, that it just depended on the person. But I was willing to take the chance.

They gave it to me the following morning and said that it should help within an hour or so. It was a pill, which meant they would have to crush and inject it into my feeding tube; and that instantly made me nervous as I knew how sick that always made me. I always preferred my meds to be given to me intravenously.

But they were right because within about an hour and a half I felt like a completely different person. The nausea was instantly gone, and

I finally felt normal again. I hadn't felt this way in months. I was so unbelievably happy, and it showed. I was definitely stoned, but I didn't care. As long as I wasn't puking, that's all that mattered to me.

When James got there, I must have had the hugest smile on my face, and he asked me why I was in such a great mood. I told him about the drug that I was given and that it had worked. We got up in the chair and wheeled down the hallway by all the nurses, and they were all delighted to finally see me looking so cheerful. Within a few hours, I was even more stoned. I felt dizzy, like I had smoked ten joints one after the other. I started to understand what they meant by not being able to handle it. I sucked it up, though; at least I wasn't throwing up anymore, and being too high was definitely better that that.

As the day went on, I got higher and higher and higher. I wasn't sure if I liked this drug. I started to feel completely out of it, and the room started spinning from being so high. The spinning actually started to make feel me nauseated again, though not as bad as before.

Later that evening, I was given my second dose of it, and once again, it completely took away my nausea. But once again, after several hours, I started to feel too high and I just wanted the drug to wear off. But it didn't.

Luckily, I fell asleep very quickly that night. But in the middle of the night, when the drug wore off again, I woke up sick and could not fall back asleep.

In the morning, after starting to feel nauseous right away, I tried the drug again. But this time, although it did take the edge off, it didn't take away my nausea completely. I again just felt more and more stoned as the day went on. By the afternoon, the room was spinning, and I just wanted the effects to wear off. I was too high, and it was actually making me feel sick as well as paranoid. I started throwing up again, and my mom suggested that I take another dose of it. I shook my head "no," saying that I didn't want to take anymore, but she didn't understand. It had helped take away my nausea and had finally put me in a good mood so she didn't get why I didn't want it anymore. I didn't care. I decided I could not handle it. I was way too messed up, and I didn't want to feel that out of it again. So the meds were stopped.

Every so often when I seemed sicker than usual, my family or a nurse would suggest trying a dose again, but I refused every time. I did not want it ever again, and even thinking about being on it now makes me feel sick to my stomach.

The following week, I started to improve drastically; one day, I was slightly able to wave my hands and on April 17, *Day 55*, I was able to lift my arm up and off the bed. It happened completely out of nowhere. I was just trying to move my fingers, and all of a sudden, my arm shot up off the bed. I had no control over the weight of my arm, and when my mom videotaped me, and I did it again, this time my arm fell off the bed. My mom stopped recording and quickly checked to see if I was OK. I just laughed. I found it funny. James was at his parents' for dinner, so my mom sent him the videotape of my arm moving, and James wrote back that he was on his way. He was so excited for me, but yet again, I was pretty nauseated and didn't care all that much.

I started lifting my head off the bed on Day 56, and by Day 61 I was completely able to hold up my head on my own, even on the lift transfers to the chair. Every day was like a workout for my lungs; between Pressure Support, NIF testing, and Speaking Valve Trials, I constantly felt out of breath. I was now up to doing sixteen hours of Pressure Support a day, my NIFs were at around minus twenty, and I was still able to go ten whole minutes without the ventilator.

When I look back on those hard days, I actually do remember a few good memories. I remember the day my girlfriend who had just had her baby came in, and when she held him above my bed, he looked in my eyes and smiled, and it melted my heart. His mother was so excited as he hadn't even smiled for her yet, so it totally made my day.

Another great time I remember was the day I had a student nurse. She was absolutely hilarious and could always make me smile. Along with my regular nurse, they made me laugh hard when they did my range of motion exercises with different accents. One would talk to me with a Scottish accent and the other with a Jamaican, Australian, and Indian accent. Some of their attempts were actually pretty good, but some were terrible, which made it that much funnier.

Later, when they weren't in the room, James drew an eyeball in a black marker right on my eye patch, so I had two eyes again. When they showed it to me in the mirror, we honestly laughed for ten minutes. So when the nurses came back in, we tried our hardest not to giggle and waited to see how long it would be before they noticed my drawn eye. As soon as they noticed, they burst out laughing so hard that one of them even fell to the ground; it was probably the funniest thing that had happened the whole time I was in the hospital.

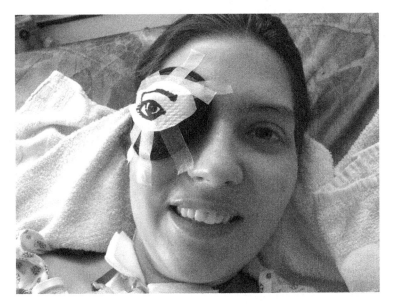

As for the eye patch, James was constantly urging me to try and go without it, but even when we were just switching the patch from one eye to the other, I would see double and get sick. So every day, I would put off removing it.

The nineteenth day of this month proved to be a lot better than the one from the month before. The nineteenth of every month was a very special day for both James and me, and I was very happy when I was able to go twelve minutes off the ventilator on this day.

On April 20, *Day 59*, my neurologist came in to do a nerve conduction test, which would evaluate the function and ability of my nerves. This could help determine how severely damaged my nerves were, which in turn could help predict how long my recovery would take. My nurses topped me up with painkillers just before he came in, which I knew couldn't be a good sign. He hooked me up to a machine that gave tiny shocks to my body, and as he turned up the machine, the shocks intensified and the pain amplified. It only lasted a few minutes but it was very painful. And just when I thought that I couldn't handle any more of it, it was over.

My neurologist asked me about my eye patch, and when I told him about my double vision, he told me that most GBS patients don't have problems with their eyes and that by wearing the eye patch, I was probably making it worse. My eyes needed to learn to work together again, so he recommended that I take it off. He suggested starting slowly at first, and whenever I did my speaking valve trials off the ventilator, I remove it then. As I increased my time off the ventilator, I could also increase my time without the eye patch.

So later that afternoon, we tried it. I was hoping to do at least fifteen minutes today. My RT came in and turned on the TV, hoping that would take my mind off my breathing so I could go longer. We removed the eye patch, which was hard since it made me so dizzy, but I just ignored it, and they set me up on the speaking valve. At the twelve-minute mark, I was so out of breath that I didn't think I could go any further, but I knew my goal was fifteen minutes so I pushed through it. And as soon as I hit fifteen minutes, I was done. I looked at the RT, and he could see the fear in my eyes so he knew that I couldn't go any longer. They took off the valve and then put the eye patch back on, and I started crying. I was very frustrated as I actually thought I would be able to go a lot longer than fifteen minutes. My RT told me that being off the ventilator was like training to run a marathon; that I would start off only being able to go for short periods of time at first, but as I improved, I would be able to go for longer and longer periods. I understood what he meant, but at this rate, it was going to take me forever to be able to breathe completely on my own all the time. This meant that I would be in the ICU for a long, long time. I could only last fifteen minutes, and even that was difficult. I just couldn't see how I was ever going to be able to do it all on my own.

The following day when I woke up, my double vision was already better than it had been for a long time. I decided not to put on the patch and just see how long I could go without it. After fifteen minutes, although the double vision was still there, it wasn't making me feel sick so I kept going. When James came in, he was so excited to see me without the eye patch on and told me that I should keep it off the whole day. So I did, and after a few hours, my double vision was almost gone. I never did end up putting it back on that day, and I never used the eye patch again.

The next time I was put on the speaking valve, I was very half-hearted about even doing it. I was extremely doubtful that I was going to make it past fifteen minutes as I remembered how hard it had been the last time. But for some reason, this time was different. As soon as I started, it didn't seem as hard. Other than having to work a teeny bit harder to breathe in and out, it almost felt the same as always. This meant that my lungs were getting stronger. I was proud of myself when I hit the fifteen-minute mark and felt completely fine and was able to continue.

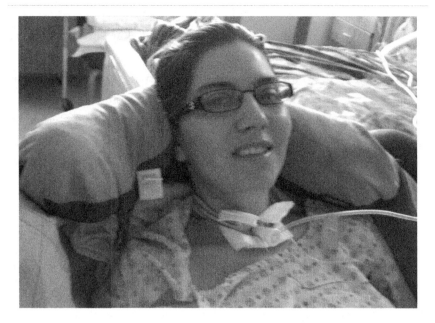

On the speaking valve

James tried to keep me preoccupied and suggested that I get in the chair and go downstairs to the lobby to pass the time. We always needed a nurse and an RT to come with us, but when the RT came in, she was someone that had never dealt with me before. She was very cautious about letting me stay on the speaking valve for much longer as she could see on my chart that I didn't make it that long the last few times. She feared that I would get worn out soon. She went and talked to another RT, the one that worked with me more frequently, and she assured her that I was fine; she knew that I wouldn't push myself any harder than I was capable of.

After being transferred to my chair, we went downstairs for about an hour and hung out in the cafeteria. When we came back, I even stayed on the speaking valve long after we were back in my room. It wasn't that I was even tired, I actually felt completely fine and that I could keep going, but my RTs advised me that if I overdid it, it could set me back. So after two hours and forty-five minutes, I came off the speaking valve. My mom wasn't there that afternoon, but when she did come in, she was so happy and probably a little shocked to hear that I had lasted that long. The RTs told us that patients generally start off slow but once they are able to do longer periods of time without the ventilator, it snowballs, and things start progressing very quickly. I was ecstatic, and I actually believed that one day I would breathe again all on my own.

I must have been in a good mood because when one of my girlfriends, who is a hairdresser, came in to visit, I asked if she could cut my hair. I knew that my hair was getting so damaged from being matted and brushed out and also from lack of washing that I figured a haircut could do me good. My family was pleased that I was actually caring about myself again as it was a definite sign that I was in a better state of mind.

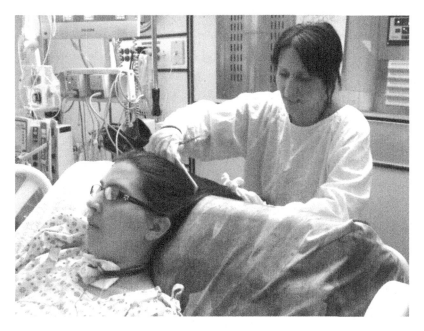

Getting my hair cut

Whenever I started to feel like I might actually get through all of this, something bad seemed to happen right after to discourage me.

Exactly two months to the day that I had been in the hospital, on April 22, *Day 60*, my neurologist came back in to talk to me. First, he noticed that I was no longer wearing the eye patch and was happy to hear that my double vision was gone.

Then he talked to us about my nerve conduction test results. Things did not look good. Although the nerves looked like they were regenerating quickly in my arms, he did not see any regeneration in my legs. In his professional opinion, it would be at least two years before I would walk again. I was in complete shock. I could not even imagine not being able to walk and couldn't comprehend living a life like that. To me, that was not a life at all. I couldn't even express how I felt. I just lay there.

Then he talked about my nausea. In his experiences, nausea was not a symptom of GBS. He implied that maybe something in my brain was being affected. He wanted me to have an MRI done on my brain again to see if anything was wrong. I instantly started bawling as I remembered the last time I went through that. I was so sick of being scared and hurt all the time that I was not ready to put myself through that again. He asked me why I was so upset, and I told him about my claustrophobia. He said that maybe I could be anesthetized so I wouldn't be aware of what was going on. If they would do that for me, then I would do it. If not, there was no way in hell that I would.

We talked to my ICU doctors about it, and one of them told me it was unlikely they would put me out for the MRI. In my personal opinion, it was just the meds that were making me feel sick and not something wrong in my brain. My ICU doctors agreed. I told my doctors at this point that I was not going to have an MRI done. My neurologist was disappointed, but he respected my decision.

April 23, *Day 61*, I amazed everyone around me, including myself, by going six hours and forty-five minutes on the speaking valve. Even though there was still a long way to go, we were actually starting to see the light at the end of the tunnel. Once I was able to go twenty-four hours without the ventilator, it wouldn't be long before I was transferred out of the ICU. My mom asked me what date I had in mind as a goal to be out of the ICU by, but I didn't know; it was still hard to believe that it was actually going to happen. She suggested Mother's Day as that was still over two weeks away, and it would be the perfect present not only for her but also for me on my first mother's day.

Later that day, the most unbelievably astonishing thing happened. My mom always had me try and move my limbs even when I couldn't, just to see if I could. And this time, when she had me try and move my legs, they actually moved. It was a very small flutter in my right leg muscle, but there was definite movement. This was such an amazing blessing. It was the answer to everyone's prayers; this meant that there was movement in my legs, even though the doctor had predicted that there wouldn't be any for a very long time. My mom asked me why I thought that after all this time, and after everything the doctor's had told me about my recovery, that my legs had finally started to move. And I told her that I had prayed. I had asked God to please let me walk before my daughter does. Although my family and friends had been praying for that for months, I think God needed to hear it from me.

But of course, even with the joy of my legs moving, that weekend was extremely challenging. Although I never felt hungry, I was very thirsty, and out of nowhere my thirst seemed to increase. My nurses and family would give me small foam mouth swabs that were soaked in water to wet my mouth and tongue, but it didn't really help. After a while, I figured out that I could suck on the swabs, which would give me a very small taste of the water. Sometimes I would have James give me one after another after another until I felt like I actually had a teeny drink of water. When I was sick and throwing up and wanted the taste of puke out of my mouth, I would have my family dip the sponges in pop for me to suck on.

One of the doctors learned that I was doing this and told me that I needed to stop sucking on the swabs right away. It was fine to dampen my mouth with them, but because my throat was obstructed from the trach, swallowing the water could lead to aspiration, meaning that the fluid could go into my lungs. If that happened, I could develop pneumonia. I was getting so much better during my trials off the ventilator that pneumonia could limit my ability to do them. It could really set things back for me and lengthen my recovery time. So I stopped using the swabs for a little while.

It was extremely tough for my family during this time as I would lie in my bed and beg them over and over and over to just give me something to drink. They would just keep telling me they couldn't because I just needed to get though a few more weeks and then I would have my trach removed. There was no way I could get through a few more weeks. I felt like I was going to die of thirst at any moment.

I thought that maybe I could have a popsicle to suck on or ice chips to chew, which maybe might help. I asked for the RTs as I knew they would tell me what might help my thirst. My RT listened to me as I told him just how thirsty I was, and I begged him to let me have something. He always compared my battle to running a marathon, so I told him that if he expected me to run a marathon, I should at least be given something to drink. He told me that he couldn't do anything for me because even popsicles and ice chips could cause fluid to go into my lungs. I was so close to being off the ventilator that it just wouldn't be worth the risk. I asked him when I was going to be off, and he said that everyone was different and that there was no way he could guarantee when that would be. I asked him if Mother's Day was a realistic goal, and he said yes. It would take a lot of work, but it was definitely possible. That certainly made me feel a lot better.

Easter Sunday, was *Day 62*. My mom had planned this huge family potluck dinner in the courtyard outside. Everyone was very excited about it and was looking forward to cheering me up. I was nervous; I had no idea how I would be feeling that afternoon.

The RTs set me up on the speaking valve so that I wouldn't have the ventilator to bring down with me, and James, my mom, and I went downstairs to the lobby. We met my brothers, my brother's girlfriend, my dad and stepfather, and James' parents. Our puppies were also there too. I wasn't feeling sick that morning so I was in an all right mood.

Shortly before dinner started, to our surprise, James' grandmother and auntie showed up and joined in the celebration. Everyone was thrilled to hear about my leg muscles moving and kept telling me not to worry and that I would be kicking my legs more in no time.

Luckily, my nurse was on hand with a kidney basin as I got sick just before dinner and had to throw up in it. She injected me with some medication, and we hoped that it would take away my nausea even just for a little while.

As I watched my family eating and enjoying their dinner, I started thinking about my situation. I thought about how I couldn't even enjoy this meal, how I couldn't even have a drink, and how I couldn't even use my legs. I started tearing up, but I tried to hide it for the sake of my family.

But halfway through dinner, I started throwing up again. I was uncomfortable puking in front of everyone and just started bawling. I told my mom I wanted to go back to my room. She reminded me that I hadn't opened my Easter presents yet, and I said I didn't care. I just wanted to go back to my room. I couldn't sit there and pretend to be happy when I wasn't. It was frustrating to watch everyone eat their meals like nothing was wrong when everything was.

On the way back to my room, I started to have a panic attack. I couldn't believe what my life had become, and it was setting in just how terrible this disease was. I didn't want to live my life like this. We had to pull over in the hallway as I was hysterical and needed to calm down, and my RT tried to talk to me. He reassured me that things would get better; it would just take time. I was so sick of being told that it would just take time, maybe because time seemed to be taking forever or maybe because I didn't really believe it.

Once I got back to my room and was given something for my anxiety, I was able to calm down. My mom said that everyone was downstairs still and was going to come up and see me. I told her no. I did not want to see anyone. I just wanted to be left alone. I wouldn't even let my dad or brothers in to see me. I had turned away friends before when I wasn't feeling well, but this was the first time I had turned away my family. I would only let my mom and James into my room. My mom tried to get me to talk, and I expressed how I felt. I was so resentful of everyone else that could walk, and I just wanted to know what I had done to deserve this. I couldn't even be a mother, something I had wanted my whole life, and it wasn't fair that this was happening to me now. My mom just listened and empathized with me completely. She told me that I was close to getting the trach out and then I would be out of the ICU.

That didn't mean anything to me anymore. So once I had the trach out, would it solve my problems? No. I would still be sick and throwing up all the time, I would still be in pain, and I still wouldn't be able to walk. It was devastating to realize that all this time, my goal was to have my trach removed and now that I was so close to reaching that goal, it didn't make me feel any better. But again, I had no choice but to keep on fighting one day at a time.

Because my nerves were starting to regenerate, I would probably start feeling shooting pains (neuropathic pain) in my arms and legs. My neurologist started me on a new medication for the pain. It would make me very drowsy at first, but only for a few days until my body was more used to it. The day they started me on it, I could not believe how tired it made me. I literally slept the entire day. I woke up shortly while they moved me from my bed to the chair, but once I was in it, I slept. I woke up again when they moved me back into bed and then fell asleep again. It literally went like that for the entire day; I would sleep for hours, wake up for five to ten minutes at a time, and then go back to sleep. But the day after that, I was already used to it and back on my regular schedule.

Early that week, my doctors had my physical therapist listen to my lungs. I had a lot of secretions from my trach tube that morning, so they were assuming that I had an excess of mucus in my airways. My PT could hear it in my chest, so she performed a type of massage. She used a small machine that vibrated against my lungs, in the hope that it would release the mucus from my airways.

Afterward, my doctor said that I needed to have a bronchoscopy done, a procedure that looked inside my airways. For this procedure, a tube with a small camera and light attached to the end would be inserted into my trach and down into my lungs. I immediately started freaking out. The idea of having something down my trach and in my lungs scared me so badly. My doctor assured me that I would be given something to help me relax, but I was terrified; I did not want to be awake for this procedure.

When they came in that afternoon to do it, I was breathing very heavily and was shaking in fear. My nurse kept telling me that it would be OK and that it wouldn't hurt at all. I looked at my mom and my husband, and they assured me that I would be fine. My mouth was chattering, and I was absolutely petrified. My doctor realized just how much this was upsetting me and asked the nurse to get him some anesthetic. As soon as it was delivered into the PICC line in my arm, I was out like a light. It felt like forever, but when I woke up, my family told me that it was done and that it had only been about ten minutes. I was so relieved that I wasn't awake during the procedure. I learned later that my lungs actually looked pretty clear, so it was very unlikely that I would need another bronchoscopy again.

Although for me it seemed like it was taking forever, my body was actually getting stronger and stronger every day. By now, when my mom did the range of motion exercises on my legs, instead of it being deadweight like usual, she could actually feel me pushing back. This was definitely a great sign of my improvement. My hands were way stronger, and although my wrists were very weak and flimsy, we figured out a way to prop up Casey's bottle in my hand. On April 25, *Day 63*, I held Casey's bottle and fed my daughter all by myself.

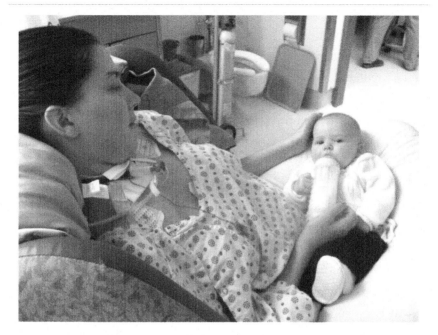

Feeding Casey

Since my hand and arm movement was coming back quickly, my PTs brought in a few different things that would help me to improve. To work the muscles in my hands and make them stronger, I had to squeeze foam blocks, which were very similar to stress balls. I remember that the first time I squeezed them, they felt rock hard to me; that's how weak I still was. They also gave me plastic cones that I had to stack on top of each other, in order to develop my fine motor movement. I hated using the cones; it took so much concentration, and my hands were so shaky and weak that it was almost impossible to even do them. I tried them every few days but eventually, I stopped doing them as all it did was discourage me.

The next time I did the speaking valve off the ventilator, I lasted thirteen hours straight, from nine in the morning until ten at night. It was such an amazing accomplishment. It was hard to do, and I felt anxious the entire time, but I still did it. I was so excited; once I could go the entire day, I would then start doing it through the night. And once I could go seventy-two hours completely, they would remove the trach. It actually seemed real to me that I would soon be out of the ICU.

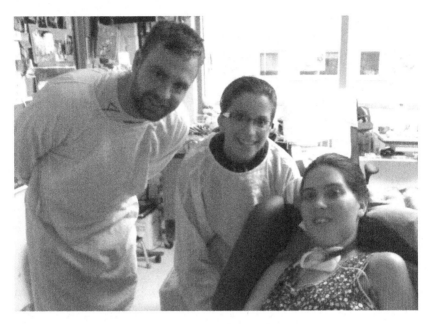

All day off the ventilator—with friends

The following morning, I woke up at six in the morning and immediately asked for my RT. I knew that if I wanted to get in as much time as possible off the ventilator, then I would need to start as early as I could. They were very proud to see how determined I was to make it through the entire day. I was also told they had a surprise for me, and as I lay in bed, wondering what it could be, they brought in a brand new ventilator. On the side of it was the name "Holly." They had named all their ventilators; some were named after Star Wars characters, and I was absolutely honored that they had named one after me. That meant so much to me as I knew that one day my ventilator would help someone else to breathe until they could do it on their own.

But out of nowhere, every little thing started making me throw up even more than before. My RTs would come in to suction my trach in the morning, and it would make me throw up. They would come in every few days to do NIF tests (I was now at negative twenty cm H2O), and that would make me throw up. Anytime the nurses rolled me onto my side in bed, or onto my back, I would throw up. Getting up in the chair made me throw up and rolling down the hall made me throw up. When given my medications through my feeding tube, it made me sick and then it was even worse when the tube started getting plugged, and they would have to flush it out with saline water. That made me throw up. It even got to the point where my family couldn't eat anything in my room because the smell of it made me throw up.

When we did the range of motion exercises on my arms, whenever my mom worked on my left arm, it would bump the hose that was attached from my trach to the ventilator, which made me cough, and that made me throw up. We tried to move the hose so that it wasn't in the way, but it didn't work. We always managed to bump it when moving my left arm, which always resulted in me throwing up. I eventually didn't even want to continue doing the range of motion exercises because I would be too sick. So we started just moving my left arm enough so that it didn't bump the hose, and I would be able to get through an entire round of range without vomiting. I knew this meant that my arm wasn't getting stretched as much as it should, but I didn't care.

My RTs attributed my increase in nausea and vomitting with any slight movement to my trach. They thought that maybe because whenever I was moved, the hose would move, and it would vibrate my trach in my throat, which then made me sick. They suggested to my doctors that they switch out the trach for a smaller one. They wanted to do this anyway at this point because it would allow for more room in my airway for me to breathe.

Again, I was terrified of this procedure, but they assured me I wouldn't even feel it. And they were right. They took out the old trach from my windpipe and inserted the smaller one right back in. It literally took a minute, and I didn't feel a thing.

The first time I felt nauseated again, I was extremely discouraged. I had hoped that having a smaller trach would help. And although I wasn't throwing up, I still felt terrible. I just looked sad all the time, and no one could make me smile. James kept telling me that I had so many reasons to smile, that I was leaps and bounds ahead of where I was just a few weeks ago and would only keep improving. I just shook my head. I had no reason to smile; I had no reason to be happy. I just wanted to die. He said that I should at least try to pretend to be in a better mood, that my mom was so thrilled to see me improve, and that it would make things that much better for her if she could see me happy.

That day was the first time in a long time that I actually couldn't throw up. Although some saw it as a good thing, I thought it was almost worse. I was very nauseated, and at least when I threw up, I had some relief. But now I was just nauseated and dry heaving. I kept telling James that I just wanted to puke. I wished that I could just do something that would make me throw up so I could feel better even for a second. James said he had an idea, but that he didn't know if we should do it, or if I would like it, but he suggested using the suction to stick down my throat to make me vomit. I was all for it. I'm sure the doctors and nurses wouldn't have approved, but we did what we felt we needed to do, and once I threw up, I felt a whole lot better.

One of my nurses asked me if I had ever tried Sea-Bands. I had never heard of them. They were elastic bands that you wear around your wrist that push into your pressure points to help with nausea. She wore them every time she went on a cruise and said it had helped for the last fifteen years with her nausea. James was excited; he would see if he could track some down the first chance he got. I didn't think much more about it; at this point, nothing had worked yet, so I found it hard to believe that anything would.

My first trial off the ventilator through the night was April 28, *Day* 66. It was successful in that I was able to make it entirely through the night without needing to come off it. I did, however, wake up sick and was given some meds to try and get rid of my nausea. Although it helped, I wasn't able to fall back asleep; I think I was just nervous and too anxious to sleep. I knew that the anxiety medication they gave me always made me feel drowsy, so I started saying I was having a panic attack and asked for that whenever I couldn't fall back asleep. I knew I shouldn't be lying to get medication as I wasn't having a panic attack and definitely didn't need it, but it was the only thing that helped me fall back asleep.

Now that I had been off the ventilator entirely for a day, I needed to last seventy-two hours before they would take out the trach. That meant that by Sunday afternoon, I could technically be trach-free. My RT warned me that it might not be done on Sunday; first of all, it was a weekend, and with everything I had gone through, they might want to be extra careful with me and wait one more day, so it might not be removed until Monday.

The first thing they would do was remove the trach and then replace it with a button to keep the hole open. That way, if something happened and I wasn't able to continue without the ventilator, it would be easy for them to put the trach back in. The button is usually in for forty-eight hours and then it would only be a matter of a day or two before I would no longer need to be in intensive care. Then I would be moved to a regular unit.

Maybe because I was now breathing completely on my own, and it was harder, I suddenly felt very thirsty again. I hadn't been this thirsty since the previous weekend, but now it seemed worse than ever. I begged my mom and James over and over to give me a swab to suck on, and every now and then I was able to convince them to give me one. They were nervous; they didn't want me to develop pneumonia, but I think they also just wanted to make me happy.

Whenever my mom brushed my teeth, she used a hose, like the dentist has, to give me water to swish around in my mouth. I knew I couldn't swallow it, so I had previously been spitting it out. But with how thirsty I was feeling these days, I took it upon myself to start swallowing the water instead of spitting it out. The first time I did it, my mom looked at me, and I had this devilish smile on my face. She asked me what I had just done, and I told her, "I swallowed the water." She laughed at my "Cheshire Cat grin" (that's what she called it) but told me I really shouldn't be doing that. The last thing we wanted was for me to develop pneumonia two days before I was supposed to get my trach out. They would wonder where I had got the water from, and my mom would have to tell them it was she who had given it to me. I was a rebel and just figured it wouldn't happen to me, so I continued swallowing bits of water here and there. I'm sure my mom figured it out, considering that I was asking her to brush my teeth seven times a day.

On my second night off the ventilator, I again woke up in the middle of the night and could not fall back asleep. I tried the nausea medication and then the anxiety medication, but neither worked. I whispered to my mom that I couldn't fall back asleep, so she said she would turn on the TV and suggested that I watch that for a while. It couldn't have been better timing because just as she turned on the TV, we realized that the royal wedding between Prince William and Kate Middleton was being aired live from London. My mom started watching it too, and I looked over at her with so much respect. It was four o'clock in the morning; I knew that she would much rather be sleeping. Instead, she wanted to be there for me and stayed up to watch the entire wedding so I wasn't awake all alone. I thought about what James had said, about how even though I didn't feel happy, I should try and smile for the sake of my family; that's all they were really waiting for at this point. I made the decision that night to make a conscious effort to try to be in a better mood, even when I felt sick.

The next morning, the RTs did my last NIF test, just to see where I was, and everyone was completely amazed when I blew a negative forty-five. I was so thrilled and mouthed the words, "I'm finally a normal person. I got the seal of approval!" I had a huge smile on my face; I didn't even have to fake it that day. My mom was so happy to finally see me in such a great mood.

I was finally ready to look at my Easter presents, and my mom brought out a bunch of stuffed animal chicks that she and my best friend had bought for me. One was a "shopping chick," in honor of my old self; another was a "workout" chick, in honor of my new self and my range of motion exercises I did every day; and the third one was a "beach chick," in honor of my future vacation that I would take when I was done with all of this.

She also had a bag of plastic Easter eggs that were filled with pieces of paper. When my mom read them to me, I realized what she had done. She had filled some out with inspirational quotes, and the others were from a few close friends who had written out some of their favorite memories of me. Some were heartfelt and touched my heart; some were so funny that they made me laugh. Even though I was going through the hardest time in my life, I knew I was much loved and had the most amazing friends. And although I did still feel sick, it was still a great day.

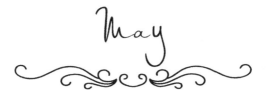

May

It was the perfect start to a new month, and although we didn't see it coming, the doctor agreed to take out my trach on Sunday, May 1, *Day* 69. It was exactly the same as when they had downsized the trach a few days earlier; it didn't hurt at all. In fact, I could barely feel it. They replaced it with a small button and gave me the fantastic news that I could probably have a drink the following day.

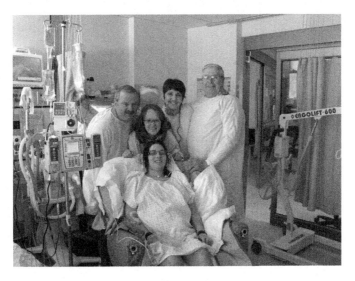

After having the button removed—with family

I was so unbelievably excited. I could not wait to be able to have a drink. Everyone asked me what I wanted as my first drink, and I couldn't help but laugh when I whispered a Sprite, or maybe Iced Tea, or a Coke, or flavored water, or Ginger Ale, or lemonade. It all sounded absolutely fantastic at this point. They asked me what I wanted to eat, and I realized that I really hadn't thought about it. I didn't have an appetite at all. I decided, however, to start off light and would have a bowl of mixed berries.

Now that the trach was out, I was actually able to speak again. Although I had been able to communicate these last two and a half months by whispering, it was such a great feeling to know that I could actually physically use my vocal cords again. My voice was extremely hoarse and quiet, but I was told that, in time, it would get stronger and stronger and eventually return back to normal.

James also managed to find the Sea-Bands for me that day, and I started wearing them as soon as I got them. I'll never know if they were what helped me, or if it was because the trach was removed, but either way, my nausea never returned again.

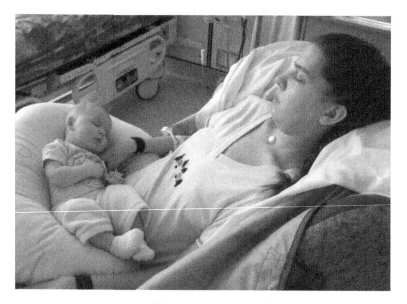

Napping with Casey with the Sea-Bands on

In order to be able to eat and drink again, I would first need to pass a swallowing assessment. Because the tracheostomy tube can sometimes affect swallowing, they would need to test my ability to swallow first. The test would be done by mixing barium sulfate, a metallic compound, with my drinks and food. The barium sulfate would show up on x-rays, and they would be able to see if what I swallowed was going down my throat or into my windpipe.

I was under the impression that as soon as the trach was out, I would be able to do my swallowing assessment. So I assumed that I would be eating and drinking in no time. I was very disappointed to learn that swallowing assessments were only done after forty-eight hours from the time the trach was removed. This meant that I would have to wait one more day. I was frustrated, but I tried not to let it ruin my good mood. I figured I had gone this long, so what was one more day?

My button was removed on May 3, *Day 71*. It was removed quickly and pain-free, and my neck was covered with a bandage. I was told that it would only be a few days before the hole would close up and start healing.

This was also the day I would do my swallowing assessment. I was extremely nervous for the test; I knew it wasn't painful, but I was so thirsty that I was terrified that I would not pass. If I didn't pass, it would probably be a day or two before they would even test me again, which meant another few days before I could have a drink.

Porters wheeled me downstairs to the Speech Therapy Department to complete the assessment. I was given very tiny amounts of different liquids and foods of different textures. They warned me that it would taste very gross because of the barium, but it wasn't as bad as I thought it would be. The speech therapist watched the x-ray machine to see how things looked, as well as videotaped the x-ray in case they needed to further examine it.

After I was done, the speech therapist told me that things looked great; she didn't see any problems with my swallowing. She would, however, need to examine the video with the other doctors to be sure that they were on the same page.

When she came back, she started off by saying, "We have a little problem." I felt my heart drop. Did I fail the assessment? Would I have to do another test? Apparently when videotaping the test, something didn't work properly and nothing was recorded. I figured for sure that I would have to start all over again. But she told me that it was no problem. She had seen enough to know that my swallowing was fine. I was so excited. This meant that I would be drinking and eating very soon!

I patiently waited in my room for her to deliver my results to the ICU doctors. My mom brought me a Sprite, which I had finally decided on, to drink and mixed berries to eat. As soon as the speech therapist talked to my doctor, he gave me the go-ahead. I never thought that eating and drinking could be so exciting. As the nurse held the drink up to my mouth, I chugged back my pop; it tasted better than I could have ever imagined. I didn't think I was ever going to let them put it down. But I eventually did and moved on to the berries. It was so amazing to finally eat again.

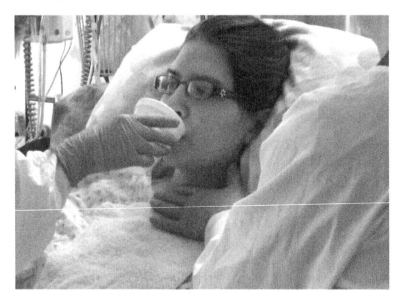

My first drink

That day couldn't have gone any better because, later on, I wiggled my toes. This meant that the nerves in my legs were actually regenerating fairly quickly. The doctors told me that I would be moving back to the Stroke and Neurology Ward, where I was first admitted over seventy days ago. I would start doing basic rehab there, and once there was a room available at a rehabilitation hospital, I would be transferred once more to start intensive therapy. This is where I would eventually learn to walk again.

I would be moving to my new unit in the next few days, as soon as a private room became available. Although we had hoped that my body would have flushed it out by now, I still had the ESBL bladder infection, so I was still on precautions and would need to be in a room away from other patients. Someone from the rehabilitation hospital would be coming to see me soon to evaluate my needs, and I would then be put on a waiting list. I had heard that previous patients had waited anywhere from just a few days to over a few weeks. I was crossing my fingers that it would be only a few days; the sooner I finished my therapy, the sooner I would be going home.

Later that evening, I had my first meal. Although it was hospital food—mashed up turkey, vegetables, and potatoes—it was absolutely fantastic. My doctors still wanted to be cautious and put me on a "soft" diet, meaning that everything was mostly chopped into fine pieces, but I didn't care. Everything tasted great at this point.

I hadn't really put much thought into it before, but I realized very quickly that since I didn't have much use of my hands yet, anytime I needed to eat, someone would have to feed me. Although I was very happy to be eating and drinking again, it was very frustrating for me to realize just how much independence I still didn't have.

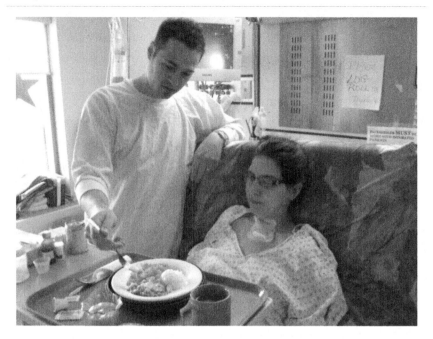

James feeding me my first meal

That night was also the first night I was without the ventilator in my room. I no longer needed it, so there was no reason to keep it there. I couldn't believe how much quieter it was without it; the machine made this constant beeping sound whenever I didn't take a quick enough breath, and now it was dead silent in my room. It also left a very empty spot beside my bed and made the room look even larger than it was.

The following morning, my nurse came in and told me I was moving to the new ward. I was completely shocked. I didn't think it would be that fast. My mom packed up all my stuff, as it had accumulated over the last ten weeks, and I was rolled out of the room. It was literally that quick; we said good-bye to the nurses we saw on the way out of the ICU, but we really didn't see that many people. It was very rushed, and I was disappointed I wasn't able to say a proper good-bye to everyone. But after spending seventy days there, I was finally out of the ICU.

As we rolled down the hall and up to a new floor, I couldn't help but feel sad that I was leaving the ICU. Don't get me wrong! I was extremely excited to be improving, but I was also nervous. All the nurses in the ICU knew me so well after all this time that they were like my family. They were very accustomed to how to take care of me. They knew to handle me very gently as I was so hypersensitive; they knew specific ways to hold my legs in the lift; they knew not to bend my legs at the knees; and a lot of them knew how to put me at ease when I was feeling scared or upset. I just wasn't comfortable with the idea of having all new nurses that didn't know my illness and that didn't know me and what I'd been through.

Not only that, but I was actually really going to miss them all. I had met some of the most amazing people that had treated me exactly how anyone would want to be treated if they were in a hospital. Many of the nurses, doctors and respiratory therapists had worked with me since day one, and many had really become like friends to me.

By the time James got to the hospital with Casey, we were all settled into my new room. It was smaller than my room in the ICU, in fact quite a bit smaller. We had Casey's bassinet in my room and a ton of my things too, so it quickly became very cramped. And we still had to fit in a pullout chair for my mom to sleep in.

As it turns out, one of James' friends from high school was my nurse. I wasn't as nervous when I realized that it was someone we knew. She was absolutely fantastic the entire day and completely put me at ease. And things got even better that day when I was able to point my feet up and down. One of my girlfriends also came in with a beautiful bouquet of flowers; as I was allowed to keep them in this ward, it totally made my day even better.

But things drastically changed when my new nurse for the evening came on. I asked for a bedpan, but when she returned, she brought back the lift as well as another nurse to help. I was confused. I needed to pee, not get up in the chair. The other nurse told me that she wanted me to get up on a commode (a chair with a hole in it that is put over a toilet) instead of a bedpan. I looked at my mom, very confused. I had never been up in a commode. I didn't even know if I could sit up in one yet. We tried to explain that, but she wouldn't listen. She just kept telling me to try it out. I started getting scared; I had only ever sat in a comfy recliner chair, never a hard, stiff commode. I wasn't sure I would physically be able to do it. I started crying and told the nurse I didn't want to do it, and when my family tried to step in and talk, she interrupted them and told them to leave as she needed the room to use the lift. James left, but my mom refused to leave. She knew that when rolling me, I needed to be log rolled, and she knew that when transporting me with the lift, someone needed to hold my legs. But when my mom tried to help, the nurse stopped her and said that she could do it herself.

When she started lifting me up into the air, I immediately screamed in pain; I still had that severe shooting pain up my thighs whenever my legs were bent. My mom ignored her and grabbed my legs and straightened them, which stopped the pain.

Once I was in the commode, it wasn't as bad as I thought it would be, but it was definitely a lot of work to sit up straight. Afterward, when I was done and I was back in bed, my mom talked to the nurse and told her she wasn't happy with what had just happened. The nurse simply said that this was the way it was around here, that I better toughen up as physiotherapy would be a lot harder than this, and that I better deal with it.

I started bawling after she left, and my mom started crying too. We were both so upset; it felt like we were completely starting over. I was scared of going through more pain, and my mom was upset that the new nurses would need to get to know me all over again. My illness was very rare, and many nurses didn't realize just how hypersensitive I was to being touched. I was terrified of physio, and for a second I even wished I could just go back to the ICU.

Things worsened as I lay in my bed. My back started to hurt really badly. I had had mild back pain during the last month or so, but it hadn't been this bad since the very beginning when I was first in the ICU. It was excruciating pain and seemed to be getting worse by the minute.

I had my mom buzz the nurse, and after ten minutes of waiting, I could not believe that no one had come yet. I was in tears. When they nurse finally came, she told us that things here were a lot different compared to the ICU. The nurses here usually had several patients at a time to care for, not just one. They couldn't come rushing at every call like they did in the ICU. I did understand where she was coming from, but I was so worried about waiting that long when I was in pain. I knew that in the future I wouldn't let my pain get out of hand before calling for the nurse.

When I asked for some pain medication for my back, she told me that she would be right back with the pills. I was confused again; I had always been given my top-up meds, through the PICC line, in the vein in my arm. She told me that was something they did in the ICU only, not in this ward. Here they delivered meds only in pill form or through injection in the stomach. I remember actually being mad. The meds delivered through my vein provided almost instant relief, and I knew that a pill would take a lot longer. I also fully enjoyed the rush the meds gave me when they entered my body. At this point, when I thought about how upset I was that I couldn't have it through injection, I realized that I might be slightly addicted to that feeling, the rush that it gave me. But I didn't have that option anymore. So I decided on the pills since being injected in my stomach was still pretty painful.

The next morning was May 5, *Day 73*, in the hospital. Now that I was able to swallow; although I was disappointed that I would no longer be given my pain medication through my arm, I was ecstatic to learn that this meant that I no longer had to be given my other meds through my feeding tube. There was no more of the gross "swish" feeling I had when the fluid entered my stomach, no more nauseating feeling from it.

When the nurse came in with all my pills, I could not believe how many there were! There were at least fifteen. No wonder it had taken so long to get them through the feeding tube. I started swallowing them one or two at a time with some juice, but near the end I was so full of fluid that I felt too full. The nurse asked me if I wanted the rest through my feeding tube, which I quickly said no to, so she then suggested that I swallow them with apple sauce. This was a lot easier to do.

Later that morning, I was looked over by my new physiotherapy team. They were basically checking to see where I was in my recovery and would decide what things we needed to work on in physio. The plan was for me to do physio twice a day, once while exercising my muscles in bed and once while up in the chair.

The first thing they noticed was that my left arm was a lot stiffer than my right arm. I was able to lift my right arm to a certain level, but I could barely even lift my left arm above chest level. This was due to all the times my mom and I had not worked my left arm because of the trach tube being in the way. I was disappointed. I couldn't believe that only a few weeks of not stretching it could do that much damage. They assured me that eventually I would be able to move it again, but that it would just take a lot of stretching.

They also saw how stiff my hands were and how my fingers were bending inward, like a claw shape. They told me that I would need to continue wearing my hand splints to straighten out my fingers. I would also need to continue wearing my foot splints, although not as often, to ensure that my ankle stayed stable. They also told me to continue stacking the cones I had been given. I thought about how I hadn't worked on them in weeks as they only frustrated me, but once I was ready, I would give it another shot.

They asked if I had sat up yet, other than in a chair. I told them no, and they said that likely meant that I would have little to no trunk muscle strength, making my torso extremely weak. When we told them about the night before, how I had gotten up on the commode, they were completely shocked and appalled. There was no way that I was ready to be up in a commode yet, and for the time being I could only use the recliner chair to sit in. This meant I would still use a bedpan, not a commode. I was very happy to hear them say that, as I didn't feel ready for the commode yet, and it was reassuring to hear that they agreed.

I told them about the pain in my thighs—that whenever my legs were bent, I would have this excruciating pain—and they attributed it to stiff muscles that would also just need to be worked out. I think they could sense the fear in my voice, and they assured me that any time something hurt me, to just tell them to stop. I didn't ever have to do anything I didn't want to, and I was in complete control of my body. I was so happy to hear that from them. I had been so nervous from the night before that I was going to be pushed beyond my limit, and this really reassured me that I would be fine.

I also told them about my back pain, and they figured that it was because of my new bed. I was on an air bed in the ICU, which was much softer, and because of my condition and my hypersensitivity, I needed something that soft again. They would request a new bed for me the following day.

Later that afternoon, in a much better mood, I attempted to use my hands and pushed the call button for the nurses. It took all my strength, but I couldn't believe it when, after a few minutes of trying, it lit up. I was almost strong enough to be able to call the nurses all by myself, and I was so proud.

James and his parents came by with take-out, and I had my first out-of-hospital food. I had a Frosty from Wendy's, and it was delicious. And things got even better, when I amazingly was able to lift my right leg up a few inches off the bed. I couldn't believe that only two days ago just my toes were wiggling, and now this.

One of the RTs from the ICU came to visit me and brought James and me a present. I was completely amazed when she pulled out a scrapbook full of Casey's pictures. Casey had professional photos done when she was just a couple of weeks old, and the RT had asked for the photos from James so she could make the scrapbook for me. It was so remarkably well done; it was absolutely beautiful, and we could not believe that one of my nurses had done this for us. I knew that I would forever have a huge place in my heart for the ICU staff.

My PTs later came in to do a full assessment on me to test my body's strength. They noted my ability to lift my right leg off the bed and were enthusiastic in believing that I would be able to lift the other one soon as well. They also wanted to see just how weak my trunk muscles were and how I would do with sitting up. I started by rolling onto my side and then the PT lifted me up by my arms so that I was sitting straight up on the bed, with my legs hanging over the side. I could not believe how painful it was. I had this instant sharp pain in my lower back, and I felt like I was going to crumble over at any minute. They noted that my spine was in a backward "C" shape, in that it was completely arched, which meant that my trunk was even weaker than they thought. After only about a minute, I had to be brought back to the lying-down position as I couldn't take the pain any longer.

After talking about everything I had been through, they acknowledged that the muscles in my stomach were probably very weak for a number of reasons. First off, I had been pregnant, which right there would make my stomach muscles weaker. Then I had had a C-section, which again would make my stomach muscles weaker. And then, on top of all of that, I had had an emergency surgery where they literally cut my stomach muscles apart completely. This meant that it would take a lot of time and effort to rebuild my trunk muscles, but as my stomach got stronger, it would be able to support my back for longer. It would just take time. As if I hadn't heard that before.

But everything did seem to be getting better. It was amazing how much better my mood was now that my nausea was completely gone. For the first time in over two months, I didn't have that awful feeling in the pit of my stomach. I felt like my normal, happy self again. And I finally started to believe that one day I would actually be able to walk again. I was very optimistic and even more determined to get myself there.

My mom definitely noticed how much happier I was and even said that for the first time since I had been in the hospital, she felt that Holly was back. I'm sure it helped that much more when James asked what I wanted for Mother's Day, and I told him that I just wanted to feel like myself again and to get my eyebrows waxed.

Now that I had been assessed by physio, I was able to get back up in the chair again. The transfer with the lift was getting better and better, and it hurt even less than it did the day before. My mom jumped in to help the nurse and gave her a few pointers on how to use it in a way that didn't hurt my legs. The nurse was amazed that she knew so much. My mom couldn't stop laughing when I told the nurse, "This isn't my mom's first rodeo. She knows what she is doing."

The chair they had me sit up in was a little bit different from the one in the ICU, and I don't know whether it was because it was just more comfortable or because my back rarely hurt anymore, but I was able to sit up in the chair for way longer periods of time. Maybe because I had a newfound freedom that I wasn't attached to a ventilator anymore, because for the first time, I actually enjoyed getting out of bed and out of my room. I'm sure it was also partly because I was getting bored.

We didn't last very long away from the ICU, and on the third day in my new unit, we went back for a visit. My mom even made the staff a cake to thank them for such fantastic care. They had been so accommodating—allowing Casey to be there all day every day and letting my mom, and often James, stay overnight. It was so nice to see everyone, especially since I never got to say a proper good-bye when I left.

One of my girlfriends came in later with homemade chocolate chip cookies, and I was so excited. Although everything tasted amazing at this point, cookies were still better than any hospital food. I wouldn't let anyone feed it to me; I was determined to regain my independence and wanted to learn how to use my hands again. It was difficult to grasp the cookie because of my strength, and hard to get it into my mouth because I was so shaky. Many pieces crumbled all over my bed, but I really didn't care. I just laughed as the day went on, and the nurses kept finding chunks of cookie in my bed.

Physio came in again later that afternoon with my new bed, much like the one I had in the ICU, and my back instantly felt better. They also took a look at my legs again, and when I kicked my right leg up in the air, we were all completely shocked. They were totally astonished by my improvement. I had literally gotten stronger from just that morning when they had assessed me to now. They knew that I was going to improve at a fast pace and suggested that every week I set a goal for something I wanted to be able to do. I decided that for the following week I wanted to be able to sit up in a wheelchair.

That weekend, I asked for my cell phone and attempted to text. It was almost impossible for me to push the buttons, as first of all, my hands were so shaky and weak and clawed, and second of all, my nails were so long. But after a good solid twenty minutes of trying and failing, I was able to punch in hi to James, who was sitting next to me, and then hi to my mom who was out. My mom quickly wrote back, "Is this James, or Holly?" I wrote back, "Holly." I was so thrilled to finally be able to text again.

I was also able to navigate through my phone and go onto Facebook. I am a huge Facebook user, so this was a big deal to me. Again, after many, many attempts, I was able to update my Facebook status to "My first update. I'm alive. Doing well." I couldn't believe the response I received. People starting messaging me and writing on my wall instantly. Everyone was very excited to finally hear from me again. And although my mom had been reading me my Facebook messages and posts over the last few months, I went back and re-read everything I was sent since being in the hospital.

I was completely amazed at the amount of support I received. I had hundreds of "Get Well" wishes on my wall and hundreds of personal messages in my inbox telling me how amazing and strong I was. It was almost hard to believe the amount of people out there who were rooting and praying for me—from my closest friends, to complete strangers, to friends of friends, to people I hadn't talked to in years.

It was so nice to know that I could now communicate with the outside world, and with the friends that weren't able to come and see me all the time, especially the ones from out of town. My phone was such a huge part of my life before, and it really made me feel like myself to be able to message people again.

Since I had been lying in bed for so long and hadn't used my hands, my nails were so long and incredibly strong. My friends were still painting my nails, so they looked absolutely fantastic, but I knew they were getting in the way of my ability to text. So I eventually gave in and had James cut them all. Texting still wasn't easy; it took forever to use my hands to type, but all I had was time, so I would spend hours a day trying to master my typing skills.

I received a message from a friend reminding me about her wedding reception. She had gotten married in the Dominican Republic and was having her reception in a matter of weeks. She wasn't sure if I would be out of the hospital by then but wanted to let me know that she was really hoping I would be. It was heartbreaking for me to write her back and tell her that there was no way I would be able to make it. I knew it would be more than a few weeks before I was home again.

It had now been a few days since the trach was removed, so the hole in my windpipe was most likely closed up and starting to heal. This meant that I could remove the bandage. When James showed it to me in the mirror, I was impressed that it had already closed completely. But I was definitely still very bothered by it. I knew that I would have this small circular scar there for the rest of my life.

Mother's Day, May 8, was *Day 76* in the hospital, and I have to say that this was one of my most favorite days. My entire family met down in the cafeteria, and James and my brother brought in a home-cooked meal of stir-fry, Greek salad, and pineapple delight for dessert. It was my first home-cooked meal, and it was wonderful. My mother-in-law fed it to me as I definitely couldn't hold a fork quite yet. Although I had a long way to go, I was just so happy to finally be getting better. I was also very proud that I had actually beaten my goal of being out of the ICU by Mother's Day.

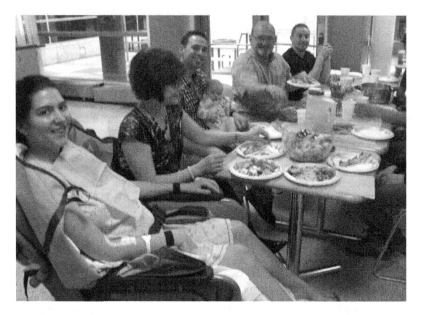

Mother's Day—with James' parents, James and Casey, and my brother

For Mother's Day, James bought me a gift certificate from Eveline Charles Salon to pamper myself however I wanted to. He knew that I wouldn't be able to go into the salon for a while, so he also set up an appointment with someone to come and wax my eyebrows right at the hospital. I was so looking forward to that day.

My brother had remembered the story back when I had drank the water when I wasn't supposed to back in the ICU, and how I had smiled with a "Cheshire cat grin." So for Mother's Day, he bought me a Cheshire cat grinning from ear to ear. It made me laugh so hard. Remembering back to that time when I had been so unbelievably thirsty, it was amazing that I could actually look back and laugh about it now.

My best friend, the one who had gotten the job on the cruise ship, still hadn't been sent out to work yet. She had been patiently waiting this whole time, and although she wanted to go so badly, she was also partially happy as she was actually able to see me getting better. She also brought in Mother's Day presents for me that included a beautiful new outfit for Casey.

It was such a fantastic day. Surrounded by my family and closest friends, I was finally happy again. I was feeling confident about my recovery and, with my no longer being nauseous, I was finally able to enjoy life again.

The following morning, a nutritionist came in to evaluate what I needed to be eating and drinking. Since I had been lying in bed for two and a half months, I had lost a lot of muscle mass, and you could see it in how thin my arms and legs were getting. The most noticeable was in my calf muscles; when I pinched my calf, my fingertips would literally touch as there was no muscle there anymore, just skin.

I knew I had lost weight, but I was so swollen in my face and stomach with all the medications that I didn't think it was that much. I didn't realize the extent of it until I was weighed and found out that I had lost thirty pounds over the last few months. I had come into the hospital shortly after having Casey, which meant that I still had some baby weight to lose anyway. So the nice thing was that although I had lost thirty pounds, I only needed to regain fifteen to be back to what I weighed before Casey.

I had some blood work taken to see what nutrients I would need to add to my diet. I absolutely hated having my arm poked. It seems funny to me now that I had gone through the most pain I could ever imagine, and I couldn't even handle a tiny needle poke in the arm. I guess I was just so terrified of going through more pain that even the smallest thing scared me.

My blood work revealed that I was extremely low on potassium and magnesium because of having been tubefed for so long. I would need to take supplements to bring my levels back to normal. The nutritionist set me up with pills for the potassium, but I would need to be hooked up to an IV every day for the magnesium. She also put me on a protein powder twice a day to build back my muscle and gain weight. She also pointed out that I should be able to enjoy alcohol again and to talk to my doctor about it to make sure.

That afternoon, the doctors from the rehabilitation hospital came to assess me. They first checked me over to see if it would be suitable for me to go there and then they tested my strength to see where I was in my recovery. They did the same tests that all the neurologists had been doing since Day 1, which included having me push and pull with different parts of my body to see how strong I was getting. They also tested my hypersensitivity by touching my feet with their finger tips. I was amazed that it still felt like someone was taking a knife to my skin.

When they were done testing everything, they told me that I would be a great candidate for the hospital and that I would be placed on a waiting list. They couldn't predict when a room would be available, but they guessed that it would be a matter of weeks. And although a few weeks sounded very far away, they assured me that this was a good thing. I still needed to get a bit stronger before starting rehab and also a little bit better healthwise, seeing that I was still on a lot of medication.

They talked a little bit about the hospital, about how I would be in a private room as I still had the ESBL bladder infection, and about the therapy that I would receive there. They also told me that someone would set me up with things I would need around my house once I was home—things such as lifts for the stairs, ramps for getting in and out of my house, a seat for my bathtub to shower in, and any other equipment I might need. This was a little confusing to me. I was always under the impression that I would eventually be back to normal. The way they were talking, I would be in a wheelchair when I was at home. But the doctor was quick to point out that just because I went home in a wheelchair, it didn't mean that I would stay in one; it just meant that most people recovering from GBS chose to leave before they were totally back to normal and finish their recovery at home.

My mom again asked me what I had in mind for when I wanted to be home by. It was the second week of May, so I figured that if it took a couple of weeks to get into rehab and a couple of weeks of therapy, then I could be out by the third week of June. James' birthday and our "dating" anniversary was June 19, so I set my goal to be out of the hospital and back home with my family by that day.

I couldn't believe how much stronger I was getting every day. I was finally able to move both my legs completely. I was also able to wrap my arms around Casey and hold her in bed with me to cuddle. It had been impossible to focus my attention on her in the past few months; I had been so distracted by my nausea, my pain, and my overall struggle that I could barely give her the time of day. Now, with nothing but free time, I finally felt like we could bond.

I was amazed at how fast she was growing and how smart she was getting. I was thrilled that I was able to see her developing, like when she held her bottle for the first time. My doctor also noticed all the new things she was doing and said that the two of us would learn everything together. We would learn how to use our hands, how to hold things, how to sit up, how to stand, and eventually how to walk. It was comforting to realize that I wasn't the only one that had to learn it all.

My stepfather had bought Casey a balloon for her bassinet for her to look at while in the ICU, and he had come up with the idea to tie it to her foot so that she could kick it. It was absolutely amazing to watch her figure out that when she kicked, the balloon moved, so she would kick as hard as she could, over and over. We were even more amazed when she played with the balloon for over an hour in her bassinet.

With everything we had gone through, we couldn't have asked for a better baby. It was like she knew that she needed to be on her best behavior as there was no way James would have been able to handle a colicky baby on top of everything else. She rarely cried and was completely content with all the different people holding her at the hospital. I loved being able to cuddle with her, and I would kiss her over and over again. I felt like I finally had my baby girl.

On May 10, Day 78, the Tuesday of my first full week in the new ward, my physio team asked me if I wanted to try sitting up in a wheelchair. I was hesitant; I had set my goal to be up in one by the end of the week and didn't expect it to happen this soon. They assured me that they thought I was ready. So I went for it.

Instead of being lifted into the recliner, I was lifted right into the wheelchair. It was a lot different—a lot more work on my abs to sit upright and a lot harder on my back—seeing that I didn't have a comfy cushion behind me anymore. I didn't last as long in the wheelchair as I did in the other chair, but as the days went on, my body got used to it, and eventually it felt completely normal. I tried to pull the wheels to maneuver the wheelchair around, but I wasn't strong enough to even move the wheels with my hands.

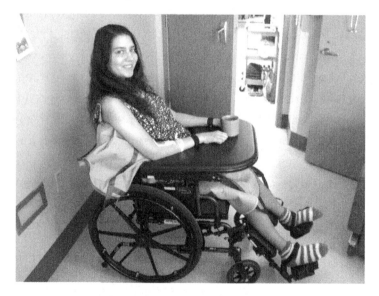

First time up in a wheelchair

My PTs were so happy to see me reach my first goal. They suggested that I set a new one for the week, and we decided together that it would be for me to transfer my body right from the wheelchair straight to the bed, instead of using a lift to move.

Now that I was in a wheelchair, I had my mom push me into the bathroom in front of the mirror. When I saw myself for the first time, I didn't see myself at all. I looked completely different; my eyes were sunken in, my skin was pale, and my eyebrows were beyond out of control. My hair was greasy and messy, and to top it all off, I had this disgusting scar on my neck. It looked like a cigarette burn on my throat, only bigger. I didn't feel like myself at all. However, I was truly happy for how much better I was these days, and I chose to push it to the back of my mind and focus on something far more important—my recovery.

On that same day, although my wrists were flimsy and weak, I was able to drink from a cup without help from anyone else. The nurses documented all of my progress, and word traveled fast whenever I did something new. It felt really good to have nurses coming to congratulate me on being able to drink out of a cup and for being up in a wheelchair now.

My neurologists came in to see me every day now to answer any questions we had and to help us out with whatever we needed. The neurologist that had seen me in the ICU noticed my mood right away and was glad to see me looking optimistic and happier. He did, however, point out that just because I was feeling happier these days, it didn't mean that I was ready to come off the antidepressants just yet. Not only would it not be a good idea to just drop it completely, but also the medication was helping with my neuropathy pain that was causing my hypersensitivity. So I would stay on the antidepressants for the meantime.

I asked him about having alcohol, and he told me that it would be fine. He actually recommended that I do anything that would make me feel like myself again. The more things I did that made me feel normal, the happier I would be. Eventually, I would even be given day passes, then weekend passes, where I would be allowed to go home. I was so excited that day that I told my family that I actually felt like "Life was getting back to normal."

My neurologist also told me that my potassium and magnesium levels were increasing, so I would no longer need the supplements intravenously. This meant that I didn't need the PICC line catheter in the vein in my arm anymore, and they said that they would remove it in the next few days. Now that I was eating, drinking, and taking meds all by mouth, I asked when my feeding tube would be removed from my stomach. He told me that any surgeon could remove it, but because of the complications that had resulted in my emergency surgery earlier, they thought the surgeon that had performed the original procedure should be the one to remove it. They just wanted to be extra careful with me and ensure that it was done right. So whenever that doctor was available, it would be removed.

My days fell into a routine quite quickly, and again time seemed to go by very slowly. I would start off my mornings by eating breakfast, and with the help of this fancy cutlery, I was able to hold my fork and feed myself. The cutlery handles were large and round, which made it easier for me to grip. Eating was messy, and I felt like a child, but it was comforting to know that I could do it by myself.

Breakfast was sometimes followed by a sponge bath. The sponge baths were very different from the ones in the ICU. In the ICU, they used hot water and soap and warm washcloths. They were done every single day. In this ward, they were only done if the nurses had time. Here, they used warm wipes to wipe me down.

After wiping me down, my PTs would come in for my morning physiotherapy. We would do different exercises, where I would push their hands with my arms and legs using different muscles. It was very tough and felt like a very rigorous workout. I was still extremely weak and was shocked that even the tiniest movements were still very hard for me to do.

But even though the workouts were hard, I enjoyed them fully. First of all, I absolutely loved my physiotherapists. They were so caring and had a great sense of humor. They always made me smile and laugh. On top of that, they always stretched me out, and afterward I felt so much better and much more relaxed.

After physio, my mom and I would usually watch the music video countdown on TV, and it was funny how the exact same videos were played every single day I was there. *Born This Way* by Lady Gaga, *E. T.* by Katy Perry, *Rolling in the Deep* by Adele, and *Get on the Floor* by Jennifer Lopez were all in the top ten at that time, and these songs will remind me forever of my time in this ward.

I was now having my hair washed every few days, but only because my mom would do it for me. The nurses didn't have the time. My mom figured out a way to lean my chair back so that my head was leaning right into the shower. It was a lot easier than the basin we had been using in the ICU.

James and Casey would arrive just before lunch. James and my mom would help as I was lifted into the chair, where I would have lunch, again with help from the special tools.

While up in the wheelchair, my mom would try to brush out my hair that was so tangled from constantly lying on it. At one point, my mom wasn't sure if she would be able to get out some of the tangles that had been there since the beginning. It was so tangled at the nape of my neck that she told me that we might need to cut it out. Luckily, my best friend gave it a try, and after over an hour of combing, my hair was finally completely smooth.

Now that I was up in a wheelchair, we started going for outings almost every afternoon. My first trip outside and around the hospital grounds was a blast; it was a very windy day, and we laughed the entire time as James and my mom struggled to push me uphill against the wind. I looked around at the cars driving by and wondered what they thought when they saw me. I actually felt slightly embarrassed. I wanted to look normal, but I knew I didnt.

I couldn't believe how green everything was getting. It was starting to look like summer. I had been admitted in the dead of winter; there had been so much snow that I couldn't believe that I had just skipped through two seasons.

After our outings, we would return to my room to do more physio while still up in the chair to work different muscles. Every day that I did the exercises, they became easier. I was even able to move the wheels on the wheelchair with my arms now. However, it was quite funny because my right arm was way stronger, so when I turned the wheels with my arms, I didn't go forward, the wheelchair would simply turn to the right and I would go in a complete circle.

Once I was lifted back into bed, Casey would lie in my arms. I loved cuddling with her. I hadn't been able to do this with her since she was just three weeks old. She was just starting to giggle, and it was hilarious to hear her laugh for the first time.

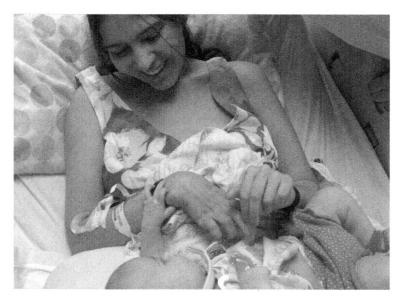

Casey and me

Later, I would have dinner, which still consisted of soft food and protein powder. I also had a large list of exercises to do on my own, so in the evenings we would work on those.

I was no longer on a sleeping pill, so I found it difficult to fall asleep. For one, I have always slept curled up on my side, but with not being able to move much, I was stuck on my back. I was also still wearing my hand splints at night to help straighten my fingers, and lying with my arms straight at my side was very uncomfortable. Then on top of that, although I knew I was getting better, I constantly worried about my future and the challenges I would face. I was feeling good these days, but I couldn't help but stress about it.

I eventually started counting to try and help me to shut my mind off, and I found that it actually helped me fall asleep. I would count to a hundred, and after a few nights, I rarely made it to fifty.

My brother was back in town from work, this time for a while, and we would spend many nights watching the NHL playoffs in my room. I was still doing my range of motion exercises in the mornings and evenings, and my brother always helped me with them.

One night, out of the blue, my brother mentioned his interest in one of my girlfriends. She came to the hospital quite often to visit me, so they were seeing each other a lot more often. I immediately had my guard up. I didn't want to see my brother get hurt, so I didn't want him to pursue things in case she didn't feel the same way back. But when he told me that they had actually been hanging out a lot lately, as more than friends, I let my guard down, and I was so happy for them. I could actually see the two of them being perfect for each other. It was nice to finally have some good news in our family.

My new goal for the week was to learn how to transfer from my wheelchair to my bed. If I could master this, I would no longer need to use the lift. I would also be able to transfer from my chair to a commode that went over the toilet, so I would no longer need to use a bedpan either. The first step toward transferring involved me shuffling my body onto a board and then pivoting from the board onto the bed.

It sounded easy, but when I went for it, it was impossible. Although I could move my legs, I couldn't move my torso very well, and my body was deadweight. My PTs saw that I wasn't able to move my body weight by myself and helped lift me to the bed. They decided that I wasn't strong enough to do this quite yet. They helped lift me back into my wheelchair, and for now we would keep using the lift.

When I got back to my room, I was devastated. This was the first big thing I had tried to do, and I had failed. I couldn't believe how hard the transfer was to even try and do. I couldn't see how one day I was supposed to handle standing, let alone walking, if I couldn't even do this. I started crying and just couldn't stop. Everything just felt too hard; I just wanted to be able to walk again. I just wanted to have my life back. The transfer was impossible to do, and I knew that in rehab, I would have to do a lot harder things than that. I was terrified of going and didn't think I would be able to do any of it.

After a good long cry, and good talk with my mom, I realized that I needed to take one day at a time. When I was doing my breathing trials off the ventilator in the ICU, I had also struggled to understand how I would ever be able to breathe completely on my own. And look where I was now. Although it would take a lot of hard work, and mostly time, I knew that eventually I would get there. I just needed to focus on one thing at a time. I needed to stop thinking about the things I would have to do in the future and instead focus on what I was trying to accomplish now.

Then, out of nowhere, I struggled to urinate again. Although I felt like I had to pee so badly, when it came down to it, I just couldn't go. Maybe it was the bladder infection I had. Or maybe it was the catheter I had in me for several weeks. Either way, I almost cried when I realized this meant I would have to have another in-and-out catheter done. It was one of the most painful things I had ever experienced in my life, and I was terrified.

When the nurses performed the procedure this time, it was a lot less painful than what I had remembered. It wasn't comfortable, and it wasn't pleasant, but it wasn't excruciating like before. Even the slightest touch used to hurt me, but now that I was getting better, I must have not been as hypersensitive anymore. Still, luckily, I only had to have the in-and-out done this one time, and things with my bladder went completely back to normal after this.

I had been sent a Guillain-Barré handbook by the GBS Foundation quite some time ago and was finally interested in reading up on it. Although I had been told a lot about the illness, there were still tons of information that I didn't know about.

When I read it, I was surprised to learn that the disease actually affected, on average, one to two out of every one hundred thousand people a year. That meant that in a city the size of Edmonton, there would be about ten people a year that would get it. I was very surprised that it was that high.

I was also taken aback by the statistics of how many people are intubated on a ventilator, but for the opposite reason. It was a very low number. I was disappointed that I had to be one of those numbers. I then read that many GBS patients have residual symptoms, meaning that some of their symptoms never go away. Most of these symptoms are mild; however, some are more severe. And in rare cases, some patients don't ever recover completely. Some are never able to walk again and are left in wheelchairs. I knew that the odds of my being able to walk again were extremely high, but when I thought about how severe my case had been, I couldn't help but wonder if I would actually walk again.

I still, however, continued on with my recovery. I was getting stronger and stronger every single day. My mom suggested that I try stacking the cones on top of each other. I hesitated. I hated those cones. It was really hard to do and frustrated me every time.

But when I went to stack the first cone, I was amazed to find that there was no problem. I continued stacking one cone after another like it was nothing. It was extremely easy. My hands were so much stronger than before.

Although my hands were still clawed, I was now able to do a lot more. I was able to clutch Casey's soother and put it in her mouth. I could hold my toothbrush and brush my own teeth. I had just enough strength to push the buttons that raised and lowered the head of the bed, and I could even change the channel on the TV. I was slowly regaining my independence. I was starting to really feel like myself again.

My mom definitely felt that I was getting back to my old self when I started asking her to do my makeup for me. Although I still didn't feel like I looked like myself, it was a start. My mom had also started buying cheap sun dresses for me to wear a few weeks prior. I always felt warmer than everyone else and too hot to wear normal clothes. My mom cut the backs of the dresses so that they were easy to get on and off. At least they were cuter than hospital gowns.

We took our first stroll off the hospital grounds over to Tim Horton's on May 12, *Day 80*. The first thing I noticed on the way there was that it was impossible to go over the curb in a wheelchair. We actually had to travel farther down the sidewalk to find a curb ramp in order to cross any street. Once we got to Timmy's, I couldn't believe how hard it was to fit through the door with my wheelchair. I started to think about how much harder life was in a wheelchair and really felt for the people that had to deal with this on a regular basis. I had my first French Vanilla coffee there, and even though the trip there was hard, I couldn't wait to come back again.

That day was also the day they removed the PICC line from my arm. As usual, I was extremely nervous and scared that it would hurt. But a specially trained nurse would remove it, and she assured me that it wouldn't hurt at all. She started to pull out the catheter from my arm, and she was right. It was completely painless, but I was shocked to see how long the tube was. She told me that the catheter had gone all the way up to my heart. After a few minutes, it was completely out, and I was amazed that this thing, which was over thirty centemetres long, had been in my body without me even feeling it. I was so happy to have it gone. I was "Pickless." Now there was only the feeding tube to come out and then I would finally be free of catheters and tubes.

That night, my mom showed me all of the pictures and videos she had taken over the last few months. I knew that she had recorded me many times, but I didn't realize how often. There were so many pictures and videos of me; many times, I wasn't even aware that she was taking them. I couldn't believe my eyes when I saw just how horrible I looked in the beginning. When I watched videos of me completely paralyzed and then of me struggling to even move my fingers, I couldn't believe how far I'd come. I watched myself on the breathing trials, struggling to breathe. It was at this point that I realized just how much I had actually improved. All those times that I had told my family that I just wanted to get better, I didn't realize that I was getting better. I just didn't see it then. I had improved so much, and I was still improving every single day.

When the doctor was available to remove my feeding tube, I was surprised to learn that the procedure would be done right in my room and not in an operating room. But the nurses assured me that it would be very, very fast and only take a minute. When the doctor came in, I asked him if it would hurt, and he flat out told me, "Yes." I was surprised at his honesty. He added that although it would be extremely painful, it would be very fast.

Once I was ready, he literally grabbed the end of the tube and yanked as hard as he could. I screamed at the top of my lungs. It was so painful, but only for a second; that's how long it took to pull out, and once it was out, the pain stopped. I sat there in shock at how excruciating that just was. It felt like I had been stabbed from the inside out. I was happy it was done and over with. I was now completely tubeless. No more catheters!

I was again very surprised when they covered up the hole with a bandage. No stitches, no glue, nothing. Apparently, the hole would close and heal on its own. I knew that since the tube had gone all the way into my stomach, I would have yet another scar on my body.

One night, when James and I were alone, we started talking about everything I had been through. I asked him about the early stages when I was first in the hospital as this was the most vague to me. He filled in the gaps for me and told me stories that I had no recollection of. Then he told me about the surgery, from his point of view. He told me about the time when the doctors had said they weren't sure if I would make it through the surgery.

He told me about the phone call he had made to his parents, and how he could barely make out the words to tell his dad. Hearing what he had gone through made me start crying. I couldn't even imagine what he must have felt, knowing that he might lose his wife, the mother of his newborn daughter; knowing that he might have to raise our child all on his own. We both started crying; talking about me almost dying was a lot to handle. I was so happy to be able to say to him, "It's all going to be OK now. I made it."

We then talked about my recovery and how much I was improving every day. I was able to wheel from the hall into my room that day, which was a huge step toward more independence. I would hopefully soon be able to move the wheelchair completely on my own.

I told James my fears about having residual symptoms. I started crying again and asked him what we were going to do if I couldn't walk again. How would we live our lives like that? How could I be a mother like that? He had the best answer and said, "If that happens, we will deal with it, and we will be fine. Things would be hard, but we would get through it together." He added that the chances of my walking were still extremely high, and there was no reason to even think about that now.

I was also frustrated about my voice. It wasn't getting stronger and was still extremely low and hoarse. I sounded like I had a terrible cold. I didn't want our friends to bug me for the way I sounded. James said that no one would bug me because they know what I had gone through and the reason why my voice was the way it was.

Another thing that I knew I couldn't change were my scars. I would have these ugly scars on my body for the rest of my life. I started bawling again. The one on my neck bothered me the most; I knew that when people met me for the first time, it would be the first thing they saw. I didn't want to be seen as the girl with the ugly scar on her neck. James assured me that no one would think that and that over time it would fade anyway and be a lot less noticeable. But as for the scar on my stomach, I knew that one wouldn't fade that much, and I would never be able to wear a bikini again. James assured me that I could; there was no reason to hide the scar. Again, I didn't want to be seen as the girl with the ugly scar down her torso. He was actually able to make me laugh when he said that I should just make up some crazy story; tell people that I was bitten by a shark and lived to tell about it, or how I was in a vicious bar fight where I was stabbed and cut up by a group of girls. Or that I could just be completely honest and say that I had survived a devastating disease, which was something to be very proud of.

I knew that I needed to accept them. These scars were now a part of me; they were there to remind me what I had gone through and how I had survived. They would help remind me every day of just how valuable life really is.

The day that I was going to have my eyebrows waxed in the hospital was also the day I had a new neurologist on for the week. Now that I was able to sit up in the wheelchair for long periods of time, I wanted to ask him when he thought I would be ready to have a day pass home. I knew that it could only be for a couple of hours since I had no way to use the washroom. But I was fine with that.

When the doctor came in, after a few minutes of chatting, I asked him when I would be given a pass to go home. He told me that I could go whenever I wanted. It was the weekend, so I didn't have physio, so if I wanted to go that day, I could. First, I would need to have the nurses give me the meds I had to take with me and then I would need to call for a wheelchair-accessible taxi to take me home and back. Once that was done, then I could go.

I was so thrilled that I couldn't believe I was actually going to leave the hospital. And instead of phoning James to let him know, I decided that I would surprise him. My father-in-law happened to be at our place that morning, so my mom and I had him get James out of the house and go for a walk with Casey and the dogs.

Once I had my meds and the wheelchair taxi arrived, the seats were pulled back, and I was rolled up into the back of the van. I was then buckled in several different ways and attached to metal clips on the floor of the taxi. It felt extremely strange to be sitting in a wheelchair while in a vehicle, but I tried not to think about my future being filled with these trips. Instead, I looked out the window as we made our way to our house.

When we got to the house, we rolled into the backyard and sat in the sun. Thankfully, it was a gorgeous day outside; since there are steps up to the doors, I couldn't go inside. My mom went inside and happened to find a couple of beers in the fridge. Now that I was able to drink again, even though I don't even like beer, I was excited to have one.

After a few minutes, James and my stepdad came back to the house. When James opened the gate to the backyard and saw me sitting there, he was completely shocked. He couldn't even say anything; he just stared at me in complete amazement that I was there. It was May 14, *Day 82*, and it had been almost three months since I had been to my own home.

We enjoyed our beers and the sunshine and hung out with Casey and the dogs. The puppies were happy to have me home, and Hugo jumped right into my lap and stayed there for most of the day. I tan very easily, and after only an hour or so, I could already notice a difference in my arms and legs. I was still wearing the Sea-Bands; I had been too scared of getting nauseas again to take them off, but I was already getting really bad tan lines around my wrists, so I finally took them off.

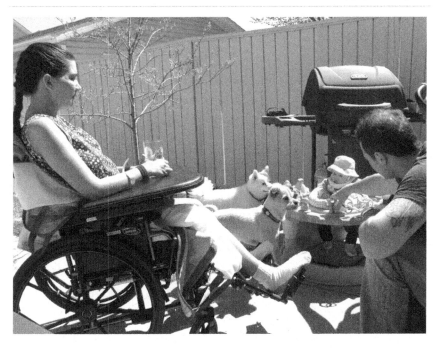

First day pass home—with James, Casey and our dogs

I then remembered that I was supposed to have my eyebrows waxed at the hospital. James immediately contacted the girl who was going to do them and just told her to come to our house instead. He also got on the phone and started phoning all our friends, telling them to come over and say hi. James then surprised me by giving me my wedding ring; the hospital had removed it months before, and I was so happy to have it back on my hand again.

Our friends started arriving, and it was so nice to see people outside of my hospital room. My brother and my girlfriend, who he was now seeing, also came by, and this was the first time that I had seen them together.

When the girl that was going to do my eyebrows showed up, she said that she would need me close to an outlet, for the wax to heat up, and that if we could go inside, it would be easier. James and my guy friends figured it would be no problem to just lift me up the three steps into the house. I was nervous, but with four guys on each wheel, they easily lifted me inside.

Being back inside was weird. I hadn't seen the inside of my house in months. And although some things had changed, others looked exactly the same.

I then had my eyebrows waxed. I was so unbelievably happy. James and I had laughed about how thick they were getting, and he had even started calling me Oscar the Grouch. This was a huge step toward feeling more like myself. I felt like a completely different person with thinner eyebrows, and I finally looked more like me again.

James made dinner that evening, and we sat outside in the sun to eat. My mom cut up my steak for me, and since I didn't have my fancy cutlery, I had no choice but to try and use a regular fork. It was hard and took a lot of focus, but I was able to do it.

Going back to the hospital that evening was definitely hard. I really did not want to go back. It was so nice to be home again. But I also knew that since things went so well, I would be given passes a lot more often and would most likely be back soon.

The following morning, when we talked to the doctor and told him that everything had gone well, he said that there was no reason why I couldn't go again that day and start going every weekend. I would just need to have it OK'd by the neurologist on for the week, according to how my week had gone. So within a few minutes of talking to him, we were out the door again and on our way back to my house.

My best friend had planned to come and spend the day with me in the hospital that day, so instead she came to the house. My mom went home for the afternoon, and James went golfing with my brother, and the two of us spent the day in my living room chatting, just like old times.

When she went upstairs and grabbed my straightener to straighten my hair, I knew just how lucky I was to have her in my life. She knew me, and she knew that I straightened my hair, so she wanted to do that for me so I would again feel more like myself.

The last few months had really shown me just what an amazing friend she was to both James and me. James had been spending the majority of his time at the hospital, so whenever she had a chance, she would come over and clean the house and do the laundry. Many times, she would babysit Casey when James needed to get things done.

This experience really showed me who my real friends were. I know that many of my friends couldn't come to the hospital all the time, especially ones that lived out of town, but she was one of the few that made the time to come in at least every other day to visit me. I felt so loved and appreciated by all my friends that supported me along the way. I was a little surprised that there were even a few people (although no close friends) that never even bothered to text me or Facebook me, let alone visit me during this time.

That night, when my mom came back, we had salad for dinner, and I amazed myself by eating it completely without help from anyone. My hands were getting stronger! After dinner, my mom and I returned to the hospital.

When physio learned that I had gone home over the weekend, they wanted to try doing a transfer again. Once I was able to transfer from my wheelchair to the bed, I would be able to transfer onto a couch, and I wouldn't be stuck in the wheelchair at home. I would also be able to transfer to a commode. That way, I could stay overnight and sleep on the couch. My PTs wrapped a belt around me, and on the count of three, two of them would lift as hard as they could while I pushed with my legs as hard as I could. They removed the arm of the wheelchair so that I was basically just shimmying my way on and off the chair.

Again, it was hard to do; I was deadweight, and it was very difficult for everyone, especially me, to move. But we did it! And I knew now that I wasn't stuck in my chair forever. After a few more times of doing it, even though it took a lot of work, we had mastered it. I no longer had to use the lift to get in and out of the wheelchair. This also meant that I could now easily use the commode over the toilet to pee instead of a bedpan!

Being able to go to the washroom on my own was absolutely amazing. I never thought that I would have to depend on someone to take care of me in that way. I was finally getting some of my dignity back.

My physiotherapists also taught James and my mom how to do a two-person transfer. They would need to do this, so that I could be transferred from my chair to a commode at home.

By now, my fingers were actually starting to straighten a little bit. They had been bent for weeks, and I was beginning to lose hope; I thought that they might never straighten and that I would not be able to use them. But luckily, just like everything else that was slowly coming back, they were too. With them being a bit straighter, I was also able to maneuver the wheelchair easier. And as I got stronger, I was starting to be able to wheel myself around in my room.

I started noticing that every few days, across the hall in the physio room, there was a class where everyone in the unit attended to work out their leg muscles. I asked when I would be able to start attending. Unfortunately, they informed me that because of the ESBL bladder infection, I couldn't attend group sessions. Although the bug was not harmful to the average person, because I was in the Stroke and Neurology Ward, most of the patients were quite old, and something like this would be dangerous for them to catch. They told me this was also why I was still having sponge baths every day; they actually had a shower room where they took patients to shower once a week, but again, because of my infection, I wasn't allowed to shower in there.

I was sad that I couldn't participate in the group sessions. I was still being given sponge baths and had my hair shampooed every few days, but I just wanted to have a normal shower. I wanted this bug out of my body. But unfortunately, because I was just a carrier and had no symptoms, there was no medication I could be given. I just had to wait it out. Every week, they started testing my urine to see if my body had pushed out the infection. And every week, we were discouraged when it came back positive. It certainly wasn't a big deal, as it wasn't affecting my body in any way, but it was such a hassle for everyone to have to gown and glove up every single time they came into my room.

As I grew stronger and stronger, one day I was able to roll all the way from my room down to the elevator. And although it was pretty easy for me to do, I still had James or my mom push me around as it was way faster.

I knew that since my hands were stronger and a bit straighter, maybe I could try doing my makeup on my own. I had my mom roll me over to the mirror one morning, and I gave it a try. It felt amazing to do something so simple, something that I hadn't been able to do myself for months. But when I got to the eyeliner and mascara part, since my hands were still quite shaky, I decided I didn't want to stab myself in the eye and had my mom do that part for me.

I tried to put my hair up in a ponytail, but because my muscles were so tight, and mostly because of that left arm that had been affected from not stretching for weeks, I wasn't able to lift and bend my arms back that far. It was so frustrating; I just wanted to be able to do the simple task of putting it up and getting it out of my face. Instead, my mom had to put it up for me.

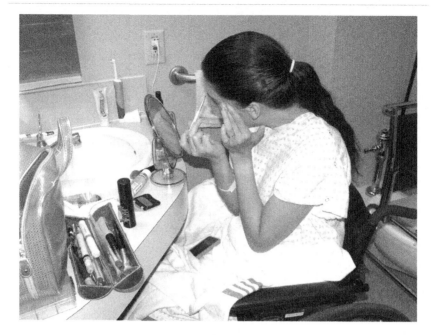

Doing my own make-up

My PTs decided to ramp up my exercises by bringing in a monkey bar that hung over my bed. I could not only use it to strengthen my arms, but I could also use it to pull myself up to a sitting position without help from anyone else. I started doing a lot harder exercises, like lying on my side and moving my legs, and it was hard to believe that I could barely lift my leg up in the air on my side. I would try as hard as I could, but my legs were just too heavy. They needed me to really work on these exercises whenever I had free time. I needed to strengthen my legs in order to try standing, which was my goal for the week.

That afternoon, we went down to the ICU for a visit. I absolutely loved to go back there not only just to see everyone but also to show off how much better I was getting. They all noticed right away that I was wearing makeup now and how much happier I was just by looking at me. I was proud to tell them that I had done my makeup by myself, other than my eyeliner and mascara of course.

Later, we went and sat outside; it was one of the nicest days of the year yet, about plus twenty-five degrees. I decided that I wanted to go over to the mall the following day and get Casey's ears pierced. I wanted to do it before she was able to start pulling at her ears, and now that I was able to leave the hospital anytime, I wanted to do this with her.

Day 87, was May 19. Not only was this a special day, seeing that it was the nineteenth, but also this was the day that I had found out I was pregnant with Casey just a year before. It was one of the happiest days of my life, and it was almost hard to believe how much had changed in just a year.

My physiotherapists wanted me to try standing up that day. They wanted me to just practice putting some weight on my legs. They first had my mom put on my shoes, something that I hadn't worn since being admitted to the hospital. My feet were so sensitive that the material on the insides of the shoes actually felt like they were cutting the soles of my feet.

Once my shoes were on, my PTs pulled my wheelchair up to the side of the bed. They had me hold onto the side rail, attached the belt around my waist, and on the count of three, I would push off with my feet. When I pushed off, I immediately shot up and was just standing there. One of my PT's was completely shocked. She thought that I would put some weight on my legs, but not actually stand yet. I stood for about fifteen seconds, but then had to sit back down when my legs started to wobble. It was a weird feeling, though; my feet were completely numb, like they were asleep, so I couldn't really feel my feet touching the ground.

I stood three more times, each time for about fifteen seconds. I was so happy that I had stood for the first time in over eighty-five days. The nineteenth was turning out to be a pretty fantastic day.

That evening, we rolled all the way over to the mall to have Casey's ears pierced. It took us about fifteen minutes to get there, but I was excited to get away from the hospital again. Once we were at the mall, as James pushed me in the wheelchair, I wondered what people would think was wrong with me. I knew that if I saw someone my age in a wheelchair, I would naively just assume that they were paralyzed from a car accident. I would never have thought about all the other crazy diseases out there that could also cause paralysis.

At the salon, Casey sat on James' lap, and I sat facing them. When they pierced her ears, she screamed pretty hard, and so did I, but we gave her a bottle right after, and that distracted her long enough for her to stop crying. The earrings, which were pink diamond flowers, looked beautiful on her. I was overjoyed that I was able to be there and actually get out and do something with my daughter. Up until now, other than the first few weeks we spent at home when she was born, we had spent most of our time in a hospital room together.

It felt great to finally be a part of one of her milestones, rather than just hearing about them. Afterward, we rolled around the mall with Casey on my lap, and I even picked out a pair of sweatpants to wear back at the hospital. I was almost ready to try wearing regular clothes again.

On the way back from the mall, we took a different route and ended up stuck at an intersection that didn't have a wheelchair ramp. We tried going a little further but didn't find anything. We finally decided to just jump the curb and cross the street. But when we started going, although we had thought it was safe to go, a car turned and was heading toward us. James pushed and jogged across the street, but when we got to the curb, we just couldn't get the wheels of my wheelchair up over it. Cars were lined up waiting for us, and finally, after a few minutes, we were up on the curb. I wanted to cry. People were honking, probably wondering why we were jaywalking, and it was stressful. The thought of being in a wheelchair for much longer made me sick to my stomach.

Although I was still getting stronger every single day, I still had a long way to go. Walking would be the hardest thing I had to overcome yet, and I would need many different muscles in my legs to be as strong as possible. I started going into the physio room to ride the stationary bike. The staff assisted with transferring me onto the bike, and I rode for about three minutes. I was exhausted and dripping with sweat after I was done; the last time I would have done any sort of cardio was just before Casey was born. But every day got easier and easier, and eventually I was doing ten minutes on the bike every morning.

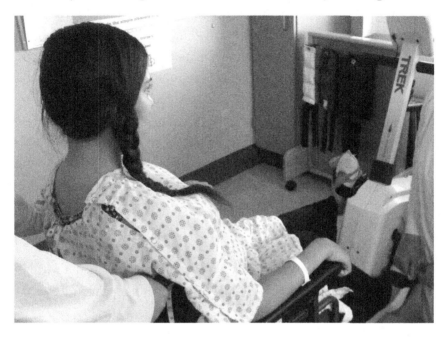

Riding the stationary bike in Physio

By the end of the week, we were masters at the two-person transfer. It was so much better than the lift. Now, whenever I wanted to get out of bed, it only took two people to do it in under a minute. Before, it was a three-to-four-person job that sometimes took up to half an hour. The lift was such a hassle that we tried to only do it once or twice a day, but now I was getting up to pee and pretty much whenever I felt like getting out of bed and into my wheelchair.

May 21, *Day 89*, I was all packed and ready to go home for the entire weekend. I was excited but also nervous about how things would go. James would be the only one there to transfer me out of my chair, which I knew would require a lot more work on both our parts.

The hospital sent a commode home with me to use, and being that my mom works for the Canadian Paraplegic Association, a colleague of hers lent us a set of ramps to be set up at my front doorstep. That way, I could simply be pushed up into my house rather than lifted up the steps. Again, I was rolled into the taxi, buckled in, and brought to my house.

As soon as we were home, I felt instant relief. I was so happy to be home with my husband and child for more than a few hours this time. When James transferred me from the chair to the couch, we were surprised at how hard it was. I tried so hard to stand, but my legs just weren't strong enough, so he basically had to pick me up and push me onto the couch. You wouldn't think that it would be that difficult, but it was. I was like deadweight to him. We agreed that we would do this as little as possible, and for the most part I would just stay on the couch.

That night, James turned on the TV and put on the season of *American Idol* that he had recorded for me while I was in the hospital. I had no idea he had done this; I had assumed he had watched it without me. I was just so happy that we could watch one of my favourite shows together.

We pretty much watched the entire season that night, but whenever I had to pee, James would have to transfer me onto the commode and then back onto the couch. It was so hard to do, and it was a lot more work than we had expected.

After *American Idol*, we decided to watch a horror movie that was on TV, and after it was done, I was terrified of sleeping on the couch alone. James assured me that I would be fine, but I was also scared that I would need to pee in the middle of the night and would have no one there to help me. In the hospital, I always had my mom and nurses to transfer me at the drop of a hat. So James went downstairs and grabbed a mattress for him and the bassinet for Casey, and they slept on the living room floor, with me on the couch. Of course, I woke up a couple of times to pee that night, and it was so much work for him to transfer me in and out of my chair. My bladder was still very weak, and sometimes I just couldn't make it fast enough onto the commode. I cried as my husband had to clean me up. On top of all that, with Casey still waking up in the middle of the night to eat, and the two of us waking up that night, the events of the night left James exhausted the following morning.

That morning, after feeding and changing Casey, James made me breakfast. He did the dishes, cleaned up, and then helped me transfer onto the couch. Anytime I needed to use the washroom, he would have to transfer me off the couch, onto the commode, and push me into the washroom. Then he would have to help me, clean me up, help me with my clothes then push me back out of the washroom, off the commode, and back onto the couch.

Anytime I needed something, or Casey needed something, he would have to get it for us. Anytime Casey needed to be fed or changed, he would have to do that. It wasn't that he couldn't handle caring for Casey; it's just that he wasn't used to also caring for me at the same time.

Before we knew it, it was lunchtime, and again he had to cook and clean up after us. I had him transfer me into my wheelchair, so I could at least roll around and be in the kitchen with him. He looked so stressed out. I felt completely helpless sitting in my wheelchair. I just wanted to get up and help so badly, but I couldn't.

James arranged for our closest friends to come over that evening for dinner, and I wanted to attempt to look like myself. I had James roll me up to the bathroom mirror, so I could try and do my makeup. It was a lot different than at the hospital. The hospital was made for wheelchairs, so doorways were bigger, and the bathroom sinks and mirrors were a lot lower than mine at home. I couldn't pull up underneath the sink like at the hospital, so I was pretty far away from the mirror. I tried my best to see what I was doing while doing my makeup. When I realized that my mom wasn't there to do my eyeliner and mascara, I had no choice but to try and do it myself.

My hands were so weak and shaky that, by the end, I had eyeliner all over my eyelids. It took so much effort for me to even keep my arms up at my face for that long that I was sweating. I didn't even end up putting any mascara on; it was just too hard. When I looked at my face when I was done, I just didn't see me. My eyeliner looked different, and with no mascara I just felt like I looked weird.

I then tried to straighten my hair, but again, it took all my energy to even keep my arms up at my head, and even more to hold the straightener. It felt so unbelievably heavy to me. I was starting to really overheat, not only because it literally felt like a workout, but also because of the heat from the straightener, and I felt like I was going to faint. I eventually gave up, with my hair in a wavy mess. I barely had the strength to even brush it.

I also didn't want to wear the summer dresses that I had been wearing at the hospital; I wanted to feel like a normal person, so I had James help me put on a bra and shirt and a pair of shorts. This was not easy. Trying to stand, which I couldn't do, while James tried to lift my legs into my shorts was almost impossible. After I was finally dressed, I felt uncomfortable. First of all, my bra did not fit me at all. I had lost thirty pounds in the hospital, and although I was starting to put some weight back on, it certainly wasn't much, and it certainly wasn't going to my chest. So my bra was hanging off me. Secondly, I was hot; being in normal clothes was a lot more coverage than just the little dresses I had been wearing. I felt very clammy and uncomfortable. But at least I didn't look like a hospital patient anymore.

That evening, our friends came by, and James prepared a big fancy dinner. It was gorgeous that night, so we ate outside, and with my newfound independence, I took the opportunity to have a few drinks. I was completely surprised when James brought out a cake from everyone that had the words, "Welcome Home, Holly" across it.

Having my friends over that evening was great for my mood, and I forgot all about how hard the day had been. We had such a great time, chatting, laughing, and drinking. It felt like old times. It was also my brother's birthday; he and his girlfriend had gone out for dinner, but they came by our house when they were done. I was so happy to be with my closest friends that night, and we had such a great time. While sitting in my chair at the table, I sometimes even forgot about my condition.

Near the end of the evening, as I watched everyone pick up Casey to hold, I couldn't help but feel sad. I was doing so many new things these days, but that was still something I couldn't do. I could hold her, but I couldn't pick her up on my own.

Later on, everyone decided to go out for some drinks and celebrate my brother's birthday, and I again felt sad. I was jealous that I couldn't go out with everyone. But I quickly reminded myself that being at home was such a huge step and that this was better than being at the hospital any day. And I immediately felt better.

We went to bed that night, again in the living room, and I had a huge smile on my face. A part of it was the drinks I had had, seeing that I hadn't drank in over a year since before I had been pregnant, but mostly I was happy to be home.

That night, in the middle of the night, I woke up in so much pain. My feet and legs were aching, like I had walked hours and hours or worked out way too hard. I also had very strong shock-like sensations shooting through my feet. I started crying as I didn't know what was wrong, but then I remembered that I hadn't taken my medications that evening. I was having too much fun and had completely forgotten about them. I was surprised; I hadn't had pain like that in a long time, but I was pleased that I knew the cause of it and how to fix it.

The next day, a friend and her boyfriend from out of town came to our place to visit. It was so nice to be with friends, and I'm sure they were much happier to see me outside the hospital. We sat outside again, but as the storm clouds rolled in, James had to bring everything in from outside in a hurry. I felt bad that I couldn't help with anything.

The rest of the day it rained, and we relaxed on the couch watching movies. This was definitely the way to go as it was the least stressful for both of us.

Later that night, when it was time to go home, I was overwhelmed with sadness. I didn't want to go back. This was the first time in over ninety days that I had slept in my own home, even if it was just on the couch, and I just wanted to stay.

When we called for a cab to pick me up, we were told that it would be at least an hour, which was fine, because I wasn't in a rush. But after an hour and a half, when it still hadn't arrived, James called back. We were completely shocked when the cab company told us that unfortunately there was only one wheelchair-accessible taxi on that evening, and it was working on the north side of the city this evening. Basically, they weren't sure when they would be able to come.

We tried calling other cab companies, but, because it was the May Long weekend, they didn't have as many taxis available, and they couldn't guarantee us a cab. After hours and hours of waiting, we eventually gave up, called the hospital, and told them that I would be staying one more night and be back in the morning. It was funny to me; I felt like a kid breaking curfew and hoped I didn't get in trouble. But it's not like I had a choice. So I spent one more night on the couch. It turned out to be a great blessing as Casey rolled over from her back onto her stomach that night, and I was thrilled that I was there to see it.

The following morning, we again called for a cab, and this time it only took half an hour. Once I got back to the hospital, I immediately started my physio for the day. When we told them what had happened with the cab, they assured me that by the end of the week they would have me transferring into a vehicle, so that way I wouldn't have to call for cabs anymore. That was the goal for the week.

Although the weekend had been very hard, it was worth it. I was even more determined to get out of the hospital and be back home, where I belonged. That day, I stood up again, this time three times, for one minute each.

I even had the confidence to try shaving my legs that afternoon. My mom was hesitant to give me the razor, but I assured her that it would be fine. My legs must have been extremely dry, and I was also still on a blood thinner, because right when I was done shaving, I noticed blood dripping down my legs. The cuts were tiny, but they were everywhere, and blood was just pouring out.

We didn't want the nurses to know that I had shaved my legs and that my mom had supplied me with a razor, so, instead of asking for Band-Aids, I covered up the cuts with small pieces of toilet paper, just like a man would do if he cut himself shaving. My mom and I could not stop laughing about it. We thought it was so funny that I had assured her I was fully capable of doing it by myself, and by the end my legs were cut and bleeding everywhere. I definitely can't help but look back at that and laugh.

On May 24, after exactly four weeks in the Stroke and Neurology Ward and a total of ninety-two days in the hospital, my mom asked the nurses to check with the rehabilitation hospital to see how much longer the wait would be to get in. We had been told that it would take weeks, but it had been a month, so we were hoping it wouldn't be much longer.

We were completely shocked when the nurses came back to tell us that there were still no rooms available and that it would be at least another three weeks. I was devastated. I was hoping to be home by James' birthday, which was only a month away. I had just spent a month in this ward, and I couldn't believe I would be waiting for another month or more.

I tried not to let it get to me and continued working as hard as ever. I decided that I was ready to try wearing normal clothes again. Since my bras weren't fitting me anymore, I started wearing sports bras. Putting them on by myself took some time to figure out, but it was easy enough.

But putting pants on was still very difficult. Without having the strength to stand, it was pretty much impossible to get into my pants on my own. After trying several different things, I learned that while sitting in my wheelchair, I would use my arms to push as hard as I could and lift up, and that way, someone else could lift my pants.

The next time that I had my hair washed leaning back in the shower, my mom had a thought. She wondered if the commode would fit right into the shower. So when she tried it and realized it would, it meant that I could sit right on that and be able to actually take a shower.

So with help from the nurses, I was transferred onto the commode in the shower. I was thrilled! My mom gave me the hose and a loufa, and I had my first shower in over ninety-three days! When I tried to squeeze out shampoo and body wash from the bottles, I wasn't able to squeeze hard enough to get anything out. So my mom had to do that for me. But when I got out, I felt like a new person. If you can picture how rejuvenating a shower feels after being sick, then multiply that by a hundred.

Just like they had said, everything was slowly coming back, including my fingers. Eventually they were completely straight again. I had been so worried they were going to stay curled up forever, and seeing them back to normal was a huge relief. This also meant that I no longer had to wear my hand splints at night anymore. So for the first time since being in the hospital, I didn't have to keep my arms straight at my side while I slept. I can assure you that it was probably the best sleep I had had yet.

The following day, May 26, *Day 94*, my physiotherapists said they wanted me to conquer another goal for the week: walking. My first thought was, "No way." There was no way that I could walk yet. I was still only able to stand for a minute at a time, and I didn't see how it would even be physically possible for me to walk yet. My feet felt numb, and I didn't think I would even be able to place my feet properly.

My PTs told me that I had amazed them this far, and they didn't think I would disappoint them now. I was improving so drastically that

I was literally improving every single day. They were confident that I was ready to at least try.

We went into the physio room, where the parallel bars were set up for me to hold onto. They had me stand up from my wheelchair, grab hold of the bars, and after a couple of seconds they instructed me to move my right foot forward. One PT was behind me, holding onto the transfer belt attached to me, and the other was on a rolling stool, sitting in front of me.

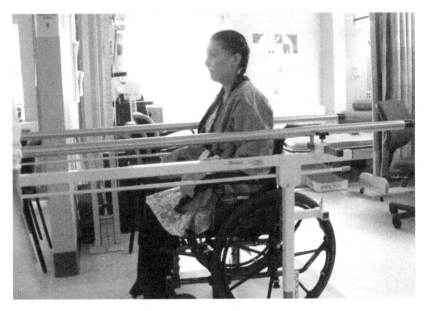

Getting ready to try walking for the first time

As I moved my foot forward, I couldn't believe what I was seeing. It was the strangest feeling. I couldn't really feel my foot moving, but it was! And then I took another step, and another. I stared down at my feet as I put my heel down, then my toes. I planted my foot firmly into the ground, then pushed off with my leg and lifted the other foot into the air. My arms were vibrating; that's how strongly I was holding onto the bars. I couldn't put much weight on my legs, so my arms were doing the majority of the work and pretty much holding up my entire body.

After several steps, I was at the end of the bars. I very slowly switched hands, pivoted around, and then very slowly walked back. My legs were so heavy, and near the end, my feet were dragging against the ground. It took so much concentration to finish, but when I did, I was so proud of myself. Finally, I truly believed that one day I would walk by myself again!

Now that physio knew my legs had enough strength in them to hold me up, they knew I was ready to do a standing transfer. Instead of them helping to lift me up from the bed and into the chair, they would help me stand, I would pivot my feet, shuffle a few steps over, and sit down in my chair. Just like everything else, it took a lot of effort, but we did it.

My PTs surprised me that afternoon with a pedal machine that I could use right in my room. It was just the pedals from a bike that I could use for either my arms or my legs. But right now, we would focus on my legs since they were definitely weaker. I could sit right in my chair to use it, and I started doing five minutes every morning. As if walking that day hadn't been amazing enough, I also finally mastered the art of putting my eyeliner and mascara on all by myself. It was physically challenging to keep my arm up by my face for that long, but I pushed through it. And when I was done and I looked in the mirror, I was actually starting to see me again.

Before I knew it, it was Friday again, *Day 95*, and I was preparing to go home for another weekend pass. My PTs had two things on the agenda for the day: one was a vehicle transfer, and the other was for me to try walking with a walker.

Physio chose for me to try the vehicle transfer first, in the morning, when I had the most amount of energy. They wanted me to master this before I left by the end of the day.

It had to be my mom's van that we used. We couldn't use a car since they are lower than the curb, and I didn't have the strength to lower myself in. It couldn't be James' truck because the running board along the outside would get in the way of my legs.

The van had to be pulled up to a curb (it had to be a street with a curb) so that the curb was level with the floor of the van. That way, I didn't have to go very far to transfer. It was the same as the standing transfer we had been doing the last few times. Both the people helping me held the transfer belt around my waist, and on the count of three, I pushed off with my legs, and they lifted me upward and over into the van.

It was a very hard landing onto the seat. But I was in. We did it several more times to be sure I could do it. It was a lot harder than the regular transfer inside; I had to avoid hitting the roof as I ducked into the vehicle, and I had to move my feet around so that they were even in the van. Most of the time, I was pretty much on the far side of the seat, half dangling outside, but it was easy enough for me to shift over once I was there.

Afterward, once we were certain I knew how to do the transfer, we went back upstairs. I assured them that I had enough energy to keep going. We went out into the hallway, and they brought me a walker, one with wheels that they could set breaks on, so that it didn't go very fast. It also had a seat, so that if and when I got tired, I could sit down on it.

When I started walking, I was again astounded that I could even move my legs, seeing that I could barely feel my feet. But very slowly, I stepped one foot after another. My arms were shaking, and I was pouring with sweat. I couldn't believe that it took this much energy to walk just a few steps. I only walked a few meters before I had to sit down. We did this about three times.

That's all the walking we did that day, but I couldn't believe how much I'd done in just a matter of days. Only a week ago, I had stood for the very first time in over three months. And here I was, physically walking, using my legs months, even years before they said I would.

My mom was so happy that I could now transfer into a vehicle as that meant no more cab rides for me. She then reminded me about my friend's wedding that was this weekend. I told her there was no way I could attend. She said that now that I was transferring into a vehicle, we could always take the hour and a half drive and surprise her. I wanted to so badly, but I just knew it wouldn't work. First of all, we would have to bring a commode for me to use since I couldn't transfer onto a toilet yet. Secondly, I didn't know how I would do sitting in a vehicle for that long. It was only my second weekend pass, and I didn't want to get in too far over my head. My mom said, if I changed my mind, to let her know.

We loaded up the van with my stuff for the weekend and again did the van transfer. Soon enough, I was on my way to my house again.

That night, my best friend came over, and she, James, Casey, and I had a movie night. She brought over ice cream, bananas, chocolate sauce, and whipped cream and made us banana splits. She and another girlfriend had made them for me one night when I was pregnant, and it reminded me of the good old days.

When the movie was over, and I was all set to get cuddled onto the couch to sleep, James and my girlfriend told me that they had a plan. They wanted me to be able to sleep in my own bed that night, so they were going to try and carry me up the stairs. I knew it would be hard work, but if that's what they wanted to do, I definitely wasn't going to argue!

James took my arms, and my friend took my legs, and slowly they carried me up the stairs. Because I was such deadweight, I think it was a lot harder than they thought it would be.

Once we were in my bedroom, they literally had to toss me up onto the bed. We have a very tall bed, so it wasn't as simple as just placing me on it. I hadn't been upstairs in my home in so long, and it felt so nice to be in my own bed again.

I thought for sure that I would have the most amazing sleep that night, but unfortunately, I woke up several times to pee. I was scared. I didn't know how I was going to get off the bed and if I would make it to the washroom in time. I woke up James, trying not to wake up Casey as she was still sleeping in a bassinet in our room. James got up, and as I slid off the side, he helped move me into the commode that he had brought upstairs. Once I was done, getting back up was even harder. James had to pick me up and throw me upward again to get me back on the mattress. We had to do this a few times that night, and in the morning I could tell James was pretty tired once again.

My girlfriend had gone home once we had gone to bed, and we hadn't really thought about how I would get back downstairs. But James just picked me up in his arms and carried me down the stairs. Luckily, it was a lot easier than going up them.

James again had to help me dress and make us breakfast, get me in and out of my chair whenever I wanted to pee, or move to the couch. But he told me that things already felt a lot easier now that I was able to do a full standing transfer.

I asked him to bring me my makeup and a TV stand, and I did my makeup right in the living room rather than the bathroom. This was way easier for me. I tried to straighten my hair, but I couldn't. Again, it just made me too hot. I felt like fainting every time I tried. So, instead, my hair was just a big mess. I wanted to put it up in a ponytail, but I couldn't even do that; my left arm was still too tight to go back that far. I felt very discouraged.

When James asked me what I wanted to do that day, I couldn't think of anything. What was there to do other than watch TV? I couldn't transfer into his truck, so I couldn't go anywhere. I started crying. I just wanted my life back. I wanted to be able to come and go as I pleased. I wanted to leave my house! I wanted to be able to get up and pick up my daughter and hold her. I wanted to be able to walk across my house to the kitchen and get myself a drink of water. I wanted to help with the dishes. I wanted to be able to pee and put my clothes on, without the help of my husband. I wanted to be able to do my hair. And I especially wanted to go to my girlfriend's wedding that night. But I knew I couldn't do any of these things, and it just made me cry.

James immediately suggested that we go to the mall. He didn't care if I hadn't transferred into his truck yet; we were going to learn and figure it out together. Then we could at least wander around the mall and do some shopping. Maybe that would help me feel like myself again.

I couldn't help but smile. My husband was determined to make me feel better.

We went outside and lined up the wheelchair beside his truck. I noticed the handle on the inside of the door and decided that I would reach for that as James pushed me upward. The hard part would be the running board because I would have to somehow get my dangling legs up and over them.

On the count of three, I stood up and pushed as hard as I could with my legs. James held onto my transfer belt and tossed me upward into the truck. It worked! I was surprised; the running boards had actually helped as I was able to place one foot up on it and push off from there. I was in!

James loaded up Casey and my wheelchair, and we headed off to the mall. Once we got there, as James was looking for a parking spot, he realized that there wasn't a curb beside the stalls. There was no way I could get out of the vehicle without a curb to step onto. Without the curb, it was that much more that I had to step down to, and being in such a tall truck would be impossible for me to reach.

James kept driving around until he happened to find a stall right in front, in the underground parking. It was probably one of the only stalls that were right beside a curb, where the sidewalk started. The chances were very slim that a spot that close to the doors would be available. We couldn't believe our luck.

So again, James helped me slide out of the truck and into the chair. Getting out was a lot easier than in. James put a pillow on my lap and set Casey on top, and we strolled into the mall.

As soon as we walked through the doors, people instantly started staring at us. I was in a wheelchair, so of course people couldn't help but look, probably wondering what was wrong with me, seeing that I'm so young. But with Casey on my lap, people couldn't help but notice us, and everyone gave us the hugest smiles.

James wheeled me over to the lingerie store, so I could buy some new bras. All my other bras were too big for me now, so I was stuck wearing sports bras all the time.

When I went to try them on, I knew that I would need James' help, but I wasn't sure how it worked. I was surprised when they let us both into the handicap stall. James helped me try on a bunch, and I settled on three new ones, two cup sizes smaller than I was before. It was hard to believe that I had actually lost that much weight.

Once we were done there, we wheeled around the mall for a bit longer and then transferred back into the truck. It was already easier than the last time. I was so happy. This meant that I was no longer stuck in my house!

We ended up going over to my brother's girlfriend's house after shopping. My brother had texted us to come over as he had some two-by-fours in his truck that we could use to roll me into her house. We spent the rest of the afternoon with them. My life actually felt normal that day.

Back at home, we again watched movies, and when it was time for bed, I knew that I would have to sleep on the couch since there was no one else there to help. But James was having none of that. He picked me up and carried me up the stairs all on his own.

I had so many ups and downs that day, but I went to sleep extremely happy that night.

The following day, while sitting on the couch, James lay Casey down, so I could try changing her. I wasn't very strong or coordinated, but I was successful at changing her diaper. It's not something that would seem like that big of a deal, but to me it was. I could finally change my daughter's diapers! This was good news for James as well, seeing that it was one less thing he had to constantly do.

Later on, a bunch of friends came over to visit. It was gorgeous outside, so we all sat in the backyard. The boys decided to go to the driving range across the street and let us girls hang out.

We spent the afternoon enjoying the sun and chatting for hours. Being with my friends was when I felt that things were the most normal. It felt like old times to be chatting, and I would always forget about my GBS.

Casey was on the pillow on my lap while I was in my wheelchair, something she did most of the time. But this time, she was especially squirmy. She was getting to that age where she just didn't want to sit still anymore. As she wiggled around, I tried to pick her up, but I just couldn't. My arms were still too weak, and Casey was just too heavy. One of my girlfriends saw that I was struggling and grabbed Casey so she wouldn't fall off my lap. I wanted to cry. I was so embarrassed and frustrated that I couldn't even hold my own daughter without help from someone else.

That night, since we were comfortable with transferring into James' truck, we went over to James' parents' for dinner. They had moved when I was in the ICU, and their new house didn't have steps into their house, so it would be easy for me to get inside.

We had a fantastic home-cooked meal, something that I was really starting to miss. When I had first started eating solid foods again, everything tasted fantastic. But now I was definitely getting sick of hospital food.

Back to the hospital I went that night. I was starting to feel like I was living two separate lives. Things at home felt somewhat normal. The hospital was just getting really depressing. I felt like I was in jail with my weekend passes.

That week during physio, instead of doing exercises, we walked with a walker. I focused on stepping each foot one in front of the other, and I went so much farther than the week before. The first day, I walked about a hundred and eighty feet around the hallways, and the second day I doubled that.

Every day I grew stronger and stronger, and eventually I could even do my transfers all by myself. I was strong enough to stand up on my own, take a few steps, and sit down in my chair. This was one of the most exciting things for me. I didn't have very much independence, but now that I could do this, I could get up off my bed and into my chair, or onto the commode, without help from anyone. To be able to come and go as I pleased was a huge step.

I was regaining so much more independence compared to the previous weekend that I rarely saw the nurses anymore. First of all, they didn't need to help transfer anymore. They also used to come in and bring me my pills three times a day. But since I was still on isolation and they had to gown up every time they came into my room and since they didn't have a reason to come in anymore, they eventually just started handing me my pills right at the door.

I could shower all by myself and could even squeeze the shampoo and conditioner out of the bottles now. I was strong enough to put my pants around my ankles and then stand to bring them up to my waist. I could dress and feed myself. I could use the washroom by myself. My arm was even getting better to the point that I could brush my own hair. The nurses barely did anything for me anymore. I was slowly coming back. A part of me started to wonder why I was still in the hospital. The only thing that was keeping me here was my physiotherapy.

June

It was June 1, *Day 100*. I couldn't believe I had been in the hospital for one hundred days. I was starting to get really bored. And I know James was too. He still came every single morning and would stay until around eight o'clock each night. The days would drag as we struggled to find things to do between my physio sessions. We could only stroll around the hospital so many times.

As I lay in my hospital bed, watching Casey as she played on her daddy's lap, I thought about how she had spent the last four months of her life in this hospital. She was here almost every single day for at least eight hours. She was growing up in a hospital room, and it broke my heart. I had at least spent twenty-six years in my own home, whereas she had spent almost her entire life here. I just wanted to go home with my daughter and husband for good.

The following day, when I had physio, it only made me question things even more. They took me for a walk with the walker around the unit, for about ten minutes, and that was it. No strengthening, no exercises, nothing. My mom and I were both frustrated; I was sitting around for hours and hours waiting to do my physio, and it had only been ten minutes long. Then I had to sit around for hours again until the following day when I would do ten more minutes.

My mom and I talked about how I felt, and she cried when she told me that it broke her heart too to see me playing with my daughter in a hospital room. She hated watching Casey grow up here. She didn't think there was any reason for me to be in the hospital anymore. She didn't see why I couldn't wait for the rehabilitation hospital at home. The last we had heard, it could still be another few weeks, and who knew if that was even accurate.

She started throwing around some ideas. She suggested that maybe I should go home. I was fully capable of living at home, as this was proved on the weekends that I spent there. The only thing that I would be missing out on was my physio. We had received thirty thousand dollars from the fundraiser to help us out with whatever we needed, and I could easily pay for someone to come to my home every day for physio with that. James was still off work on paternity leave and would be till October, so it's not like I would be alone at home. My mom also works part-time, so she would be around to help us as well.

The more we talked about it, the better it sounded. I hadn't done stairs yet, but sleeping on my couch until I was strong enough to do them sounded way better to me than staying here. I was only on pain medication now, which they gave me by pill, and I could easily get a prescription and take them at home. My blood pressure was normal; my magnesium levels were normal; everything was normal. There were no medical reasons for me to be in a hospital anymore.

I had made my decision. I was ready to go home and wait for the rehabilitation hospital there.

The next time my neurologist came in to talk to me, I told him that I wanted to leave. I told him my reasons, about how I didn't think there were any medical reasons for me to stay here anymore, and I thought that I could fully function at home until the rehabilitation hospital was ready for me.

He immediately disputed my reasoning. He didn't think I was ready yet. Although I felt like I was better, there was still a lot more work I needed to do, and he didn't think it would be smart for me to leave.

James wasn't there yet, so he told me that once James got there, he would come back and talk to the two of us about it. He didn't want to leave James in the dark and wanted him to have a say in this as well.

When James came in, I told him how I felt. I could immediately sense the hesitation in his voice. I don't think he felt I was quite ready yet either. He wanted to hear more about what the doctor had to say.

When the doctor came back, he first pointed out that to be able to get into In-Patient Therapy at the rehabilitation hospital, I needed to be in a hospital. If I went home, I would lose my spot and would only be considered for Out-Patient Therapy. He assured me that In-Patient Therapy was a lot better; I would spend a majority of my day on physio compared to only a few hours, a few times a week, with Out-Patient Therapy. If I was only able to spend a few days a week on my physio, it might take twice as long to recover. He understood why I wanted to go home, and it was my decision, but he wanted us to really think about it before we decided.

He went on to tell me that even though I had been going home on the weekends, it was still a lot different than everyday life. James was currently putting aside other things so that he could focus entirely on me over the weekends. With me permanently around, James would have to take care of me and Casey, as well as the everyday errands and chores.

He then asked me to take off my shoes and socks and then put them back on. I knew I couldn't do that yet, and I told him so. He simply smiled. He knew he was right. Although I was feeling more independent, I wasn't quite there. I couldn't even put on my own socks and shoes yet.

I realized that I had a long way to go still, but I told him that I just couldn't sit here every day anymore. I was so sick of my room and so unbelievably bored. I wanted to be at home with my husband and daughter. I didn't like it that physio was so short, and it just didn't seem worth it to me to sit around all day waiting for it. But my biggest fear of all was that I would be waiting forever. I had heard stories of patients that had waited months and months to get into the rehabilitation hospital. I couldn't picture being here for any more weeks, let alone months.

He had an idea and asked if I would be happy with day passes. Instead of just weekend passes, once I had done my physio for the day, I could leave. I could spend my afternoon and evenings at home and then return to the hospital to sleep and for the physio the following day. I would still be a patient in the hospital and qualify for Inpatient Therapy at the rehabilitation hospital.

James looked very happy with the suggestion. I could tell that the thought of me coming home for good overwhelmed him. I hadn't really thought about how it would affect him. I just assumed he would want me at home. But this idea would give him the best of both worlds. He would have me home in the evenings but would still have his mornings to get things done around the house, and I would have the help I needed during the day at the hospital.

Then my doctor said he would talk to physiotherapy to see if they could provide more therapy for me. I was happy about that. If I felt like I was doing more here, then it would be worth it for me to stay.

We then made the decision that if I hadn't been moved by June 19 (James' birthday, which was my original goal to be home by), I would go home. That was still almost three weeks away, and I knew that was as long as I was willing to wait. If I still hadn't been moved by then, I would pursue another option.

My mom and I took it upon ourselves to start looking into what those options might be. We talked to Out-Patient Therapy at the hospital and learned that I could do my therapy there. It, however, would still only be a few days a week.

I knew this meant that my recovery might take longer. But at this point, I think I decided that being at home with Casey was more important than my recovery. I would rather my recovery take a few months longer and be at home with her.

I was willing to stick it out until mid June, but I didn't really believe that I would be moved by then. In my mind, I would be going home at that time.

My doctor must have gone to talk to my physiotherapists shortly after because they then came in to talk to me about everything that had been discussed.

They had been worried that they were pushing me too hard, and that was the reason that they were doing such short physio sessions with me. They assured me that now that they knew I could handle, and wanted more physio, they would provide me with it.

Now along with the walking, I would also focus on riding the bike more, using the arm pedals for the upper body, and even start doing some leg exercises with the other PT.

My physiotherapists would also look into getting me equipment to use at home, now that I would be spending more time there. The equipment included a wheelchair, a walker, a commode, and a bath seat. They also had me apply for a handicapped sticker so that when I went out, James would be able to park in handicapped stalls, so it would be easier for me to get out and do things.

Later that afternoon, I had a visitor. It was one of the respiratory therapists from the ICU. He was someone that we had gotten very close to during my time in the ICU. He was also the one that, after I did the NIF test for him, had told us we could stay at his home in Phoenix.

I loved having visitors from the ICU. It was nice to see a familiar face, especially someone that knew me and my condition so well. We talked for a few minutes, mostly about my recovery, and he mentioned that it wouldn't be long before I would be ready to take that trip to Phoenix.

I was speechless. I didn't realize he was serious about letting us stay there. But as he continued talking about it, I realized he was dead serious.

He then told me that he and his wife had thought of donating his vacation home for our auction, for people to bid on, but instead decided to just let us use it instead. He felt that I needed and deserved a vacation after all I had been through. He and James started discussing dates, and they came up with September or October. We presumed I would be home from rehab latest by mid July, and that would give me a few more months at home to adjust. By then, I would hopefully be well enough to travel.

It was hard to picture where I would be at in September/October. Would I be in a wheelchair still? I really had no idea how long it would be before I could easily walk without help. And although my excitement grew, realizing that we really were going to get to go to Phoenix, I was still apprehensive about September/October. I wanted to be able to fully enjoy this trip; I wanted to be able to get in and out of the pool, and I didn't want to be stuck in a wheelchair my whole vacation.

Either way, I was so unbelievably grateful to him. I couldn't believe that someone would just offer up their home for us to stay in for free. I truly appreciated this huge gift to our family.

A little bit later, my neurologist came back to talk to me. It wasn't like him to come twice in one day. But he had some good news. Apparently, the rehabilitation hospital had just called, requesting my file. He said they usually do this when they are preparing to have me moved. He figured it would only be a matter of days before I would be transferred over.

I couldn't help but wonder if he had anything to do with this. I knew that he also worked out of that hospital, and I guessed that he had called over to get the ball rolling. It seemed like too much of a coincidence, that within just a few hours of talking to him and telling him that I wanted to go home, they had called.

It really didn't matter if he had made a call on my behalf or if they had called all on their own. I was thrilled. I really hoped their calling meant that I would be moving there soon. As much as I just wanted to go home, I knew that this hospital would be a great place for me to go. I knew it would be the best place for my recovery.

The weekend came, and on June 3, *Day 102*, I was at home with my family once again. I was especially excited for this weekend pass as my brother was having his birthday party on the Saturday. I had missed going out on his actual birthday, but I was able to attend the party. It was at his girlfriend's house in her backyard, which I could easily roll my wheelchair right into. A ton of friends would be going, so I would get to see the people that couldn't come visit me as often.

Everything was definitely getting easier at home. I was doing my own transfers now, so I could pivot in and out of my chair all on my own. This was a huge burden taken off James. He didn't have to continuously move me back and forth between the couch and my chair. I could do it whenever I pleased.

James carried me up the stairs that night and again had to throw me into bed to sleep. The best part of being at home was definitely being able to sleep in my own bed, but I felt bad that James had to help me in the middle of the night whenever I needed to get up to pee. It was always such an ordeal to get me off and on our tall bed, and when you are in a deep sleep, it was that much more annoying.

The next morning, I once again tried to straighten my hair, and once again I was just too hot and tired to do it. I was at least able to brush my own hair though, and ended up leaving it wavy. But I just wished I could straighten my hair again. This is when I looked most like me.

Once I was ready, James, Casey, and I headed over to my brother's birthday party. It was pretty nice out that day, which was perfect, seeing that we would be outside.

Once I transferred out of the truck, James pushed my wheelchair into the backyard, and immediately people started coming over to say hi. Other than my closest friends who came to visit me in the hospital, most people hadn't seen me in months. And seeing that Casey was so young when I had first gone into the hospital, a lot of people hadn't even met her yet.

Everyone asked how I was doing, and I was thrilled and proud to be able to tell them how much better I was and how far I'd come in the last few months. There was a time that I truly didn't believe I would ever get out of the hospital, and it felt great when I told them that I would be home with my family soon. I actually meant it.

It was weird to be at a party in a wheelchair. I sat in my chair, watching everyone move around while I was stuck in one spot. I could certainly wheel around by myself, but in the grass it was a lot harder and took a lot of energy that I just didn't feel like using.

I felt guilty that I had to rely on my friends a lot. Whenever I needed a drink, I would have to ask someone to grab it for me. Whenever I wanted to go talk to someone, or just move in general, I would have to ask my friends to move me. I had no reason to be embarrassed or to feel guilty about my condition, but I was. After being an independent person fully capable of taking care of me, it was hard having to depend on others all the time.

When I went to bed that night, I was so grateful that I was able to go to my brother's birthday party. Spending time with Casey and James always made me happy, but it was when I was hanging out with friends that things felt most normal. It was probably because when I was with friends, I wasn't trying to do things around the house. There was a lot less stress on me when I didn't have to do everyday things. When I was busy socializing, it took the focus off the things that I had trouble doing or could no longer do.

The following morning, my cousin and a girlfriend from out of town came up for the day to visit me. We spent the afternoon in my living room chatting, and it was really nice to catch up with people that I couldn't see all the time. James got to talking about all the things that had happened the last few months, and it really reminded me of just how far I had come.

Back at the hospital for the week, I really started to notice my improvements. In physio, when my PTs would exercise my legs, I was amazed at how far back they could bend my knees without it hurting. The stretches they were doing every morning were really helping me.

I was walking every day with the walker, with help from my PTs, for about twenty minutes around the unit or outside around the hospital. It was getting easier, and I could walk a bit longer every day, but it still took a lot of energy and a lot of concentration. I definitely had a limit of how long I could walk for, and once I hit my limit, I knew I was done for the day.

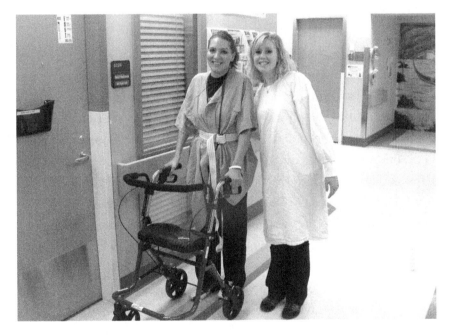

Walking with a walker with my physiotherapist

My physiotherapists noticed that as I walked, my toes dragged a little bit. My ankles were extremely weak, which made it hard for me to lift my toes as I walked. They wanted me to strengthen my ankles, so they gave me several different exercises to work on. One was for me to sit in my wheelchair, with my feet flat in front of me, and to lift my toes. The first time I did it, I lifted my toes as hard as I could up into the air. But when I looked down at my feet, they hadn't moved an inch. I tried over and over again, but nothing happened. I could not lift my toes at all.

The next thing they had me try was to stand on my tippy toes. I wheeled up to a wall in the hallway outside my hospital room, and with the help of the railing, I stood up. But as I tried to stand up on the tips of my toes, I couldn't do it. I felt like I was pushing off on my feet as hard as I could, but I didn't move.

Even though I couldn't do these things yet, I still tried doing them every day. I knew that the more I worked on them, the stronger my ankles would get, and the easier it would get.

Although I had officially only been practicing walking for eleven days, my physiotherapists felt I was ready to try doing stairs. I was hesitant; I wasn't sure my legs were quite strong enough.

We went into the physio room, where they had a set of stairs built right in the room to practice on. There were only about four or five steps, but it was still extremely intimidating to me. I wheeled up to the steps, and as I held onto the railings, I stood up. My PT attached a belt around my waist for her to hold onto as she followed me up the steps.

I was told to go up the stairs stepping with the same foot first and then come back down stepping the opposite foot down. I lifted my right foot and placed it onto the first step. I was used to surprising myself, but I still didn't expect to even move. Then I lifted my other leg onto the same step. It was so hard. I had no balance, and I felt like I was going to fall over at any minute. My PT could see the fear in my eyes and assured me she had me and that she wouldn't let go. I wasn't going to fall. I continued up the stairs, one step at a time. And then I was at the top of the stairs.

I was so proud. I knew that once I mastered stairs, I would no longer be stuck on the main level of my house. I wouldn't have to depend on James to carry me up to bed every night and back down the stairs in the morning.

But I still had to get back down the stairs. I started with the left foot this time, and lowered my leg onto the step below me. This, surprisingly, was way harder. The way my leg had to step downward sent sharp pains down the back of my leg. My calf muscles were very tight, and it felt like they were ripping.

Once I landed my foot onto the step, the pain went away. I continued moving each leg down the steps. I pushed through the pain and eventually made my way to the bottom.

My PTs asked me if I wanted to go up again. I shook my head. That's all I knew I could do for the day. They reminded me that in order to do the twelve steps at home, I would have to be able to do more than double the steps here. I hadn't thought about that. But I was extremely tired and didn't want to push myself any further.

On June 7, *Day 106*, I tried walking with a cane. Although I was still learning how to walk with a walker, they wanted me to try and see how a cane felt for me.

With one PT behind me holding onto my transfer belt, and the other one beside me in case I needed to lean on someone, I placed the cane in front of me, followed by my leg. It was extremely difficult. Not only was it hard to keep my balance, it was also hard to coordinate the cane at the same time as my legs. The PTs knew that I just wasn't there quite yet and helped me to walk. I actually made it the entire loop around the unit, but we all knew it would still be a while before I could comfortably use a cane on my own.

My neurologist came in that afternoon and told me they had a new patient with GBS on the unit. She didn't have it quite as severe as I did, as she wasn't on a respirator, but she was still going to have to learn how to walk again. She was in a wheelchair and had yet to try walking. He hoped that we could meet and that I could lift her spirits by showing her that she would get better.

The next time I was in the physio room, working out on the stationary bike, the new GBS patient came in to work out as well.

Our PTs introduced us, and we talked about our journeys with GBS so far. She had been very close to being put on the respirator, but the medication seemed to have helped her as she started to improve.

Although our meeting was short, I was glad I got to talk to her. She told me that she had seen me walking with the walker around the unit earlier that day, and it had really given her hope that one day soon she would do the same. I understood completely. Every time I saw the man who had GBS before me, it gave me the strength and courage to keep on fighting.

James had picked up my equipment early that day and brought it all home for me to use in the evenings. It was such a relief to have everything I needed right there. I now had a walker at home to practice walking with, and I started using it to get from the living room to the kitchen, to the bathroom, and back. James was nervous; he hated watching me do it all by myself. At the hospital, I always had my PTs holding on to me as I walked. And although James was there to help at any time, I wanted my independence, and I wanted to prove to everyone that I could do this on my own. So I continued to walk with it around my house, by myself.

The piece of equipment I was most excited about was the bath seat. It was a plastic chair with three seats on it. It was meant for two legs to rest right in the tub and for the other two legs to be outside the bath on the floor. With the bath seat, I could transfer onto the seat and scoot myself over into the shower.

James handed me the shower head, and I was able to have my own shower in my own home. I felt so much more comfortable than at the hospital.

When I finished, James helped me out, and out of the corner of my eye, I noticed pieces of my hair all over the bath seat. My hair was getting really long, and without brushing it as often as I normally would, I assumed I was shedding more in the shower. But when I was brushing my hair out, I couldn't believe how much hair was still coming out in the comb. This wasn't just natural shedding; my hair seemed like it was falling out.

While at home, I also tried doing the stairs. James and my stepdad had installed banisters on the wall, so I had them as well as the railing on the other side to hold onto. I had since done the stairs a few more times during physio, and it was getting easier.

But doing them at home was extremely difficult. I was able to do a few steps at a time but would need to stop for a minute or two till I had the strength to continue up. And I still had to do each step one at a time.

Back at the hospital, my mom and I started working on a video. We had hundreds of photos of my time in the hospital, and we wanted to make a slideshow of my progress. We picked the song "I Won't Let Go" by Rascal Flatts to go along with the pictures. My mom had heard it a few weeks before on the radio and couldn't believe how fitting it was to our family's situation. It was a very inspiring and uplifting song about being there for someone going through a tough time. I cried the first time I heard it. It really made me appreciate the people in my life. And I knew it was the perfect song for the slideshow.

My brother and girlfriend came in to visit, and shortly after they arrived, my nurse came in to talk to me. It had been a few days since the rehabilitation hospital had called requesting my file, but I still couldn't believe it when she told me that they had a room for me. I was finally going to be moved.

I was beyond excited. It was probably the happiest I'd felt in months. I couldn't wait to start the next chapter in my recovery. I was one step closer to getting home.

But a part of me was also very nervous. I really had no idea what it was going to be like over there. I was scared that I wouldn't be able to keep up in physio. I was also scared because I would be alone. My mom had stayed overnight with me almost every night since I was admitted into the hospital, but she would not be coming with me there. The rehabilitation hospital encouraged independence, and they wanted me to regain every bit I could by learning to do absolutely everything all on my own.

That afternoon, we made our way around the hospital to say good-bye to all the people we had met while I was there. After spending almost four months there, we had gotten to know a lot of people. We said good-bye to the cafeteria lady, who had sold us food almost every day; the woman who worked at the flower shop, who saw me ride by in my chair and watched me improve every day; my physiotherapists, social worker, and nutritionist, and then, of course, everyone down in the ICU. I could see on everyone's faces just how happy they were for me.

That night, we finished the slideshow. When we watched it for the first time, I bawled. I couldn't believe how far I had come. Watching me in those first weeks was extremely difficult and brought back a lot of bad memories, but it also reminded me of everything I had gotten through. I had made it through the most painful things I'd ever gone through in my life. I made it through emergency surgery, severe anxiety attacks, extreme thirst, and, the worst of all, the nausea, vomiting and pain.

Not only had I learned how to breathe on my own again, but also I had learned how to use my fingers, my hands, and my legs all over again. I was nowhere near the end of the tunnel, but I could at least now see the light. I knew that one day I would walk again all on my own. Like everyone had told me, it would just take time.

We showed the video to my nurse on duty that night. She cried. She called in a few of the nurses to watch it, and they cried too. They eventually brought my mom's laptop out to the nurse's station so that everyone could watch it.

One by one, the nurses came in to say good-bye and to wish me luck. I knew they had all read my charts and about what I had gone through, but to physically see my journey in pictures must have been a lot more powerful to them.

I watched as my mom finished packing up all our things. I couldn't believe that I had been in this room for six weeks, and in this hospital for a total of *107 days*. Knowing that this was the last night I would be spending here was very soothing. I went to sleep that night very happy, excited, nervous, and proud. I couldn't wait for the next morning to come.

I slept well that night, and before I knew it, it was morning. My mom was in the shower when the nurse came in and asked if we could be ready about half an hour earlier than we thought. We were all packed, so that really just meant less time waiting around.

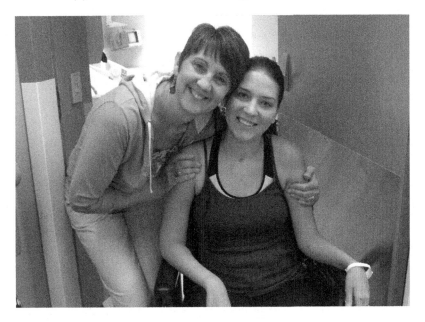

Getting ready to leave the hospital after 107 days—with my mom

An ambulance arrived, and the paramedics helped me transfer onto the stretcher. Then I was whisked away into the ambulance and headed for my next temporary home.

The drive there was long; my new hospital was on the other side of the city, but it was also rush hour. I didn't really mind. It was absolutely gorgeous that day; the sun was beaming through the window, and that put me in a fantastic mood as I lay there watching the clouds go by in the sky.

Once I got to the new hospital, I was wheeled into the admission room, where I lay on the stretcher while they completed my paperwork. Then I was brought upstairs to my new room. My mom met me with all my stuff a few minutes later.

The ward I was brought to was the Spinal Cord Injury Ward. Everyone was in a wheelchair, like me. I saw people cruising by my room all on their own. I knew I could wheel by myself too, but I had always had someone with me, so they always pushed me. I wasn't really sure how far I would be able to push my wheelchair on my own.

My nurse for the day came in and gave me a rundown of how things worked around there. There was a board at the front of our ward that had a list of the classes everyone had daily. We would wheel ourselves to each of our classes, by ourselves, unless we weren't feeling up to it. Then we could request a porter to wheel us. If we didn't have a class, we were free to roam around as we pleased. Obviously, because of my bladder infection, I needed to be careful not to touch other patients.

But before I was allowed to get up and move around on my own, to ensure my safety, physiotherapy first needed to come up and watch me transfer. They wanted to make sure that I could actually do it on my own. And they would not be in until sometime in the afternoon.

I assured her that I could transfer by myself. I had been transferring on my own for a couple of weeks now, and I was totally comfortable doing them. But no, she would not let me do it until the physiotherapists came in. Until then, we would have to use the lift. I absolutely despised the lift, but I also knew that it wouldn't be as bad now that I didn't have as much pain anymore. Either way, both my mom and I thought it was overkill.

The lift turned out to be fine, but it took forever and was very annoying. I spent the morning and most of the afternoon in my bed, so we didn't have to bother with the lift. Physio came in late that afternoon and OK'd my transfers, allowing me to do them completely on my own.

I didn't think they had believed me when I said I could transfer on my own, seeing that most of their patients usually came to them shortly after their initial incident. Most of them were starting their physiotherapy here, whereas I had already been doing six weeks of physio back at the other hospital. I think I really surprised them at how far I was already. After seeing how well I moved around on my own, both my nurse and my physiotherapist mentioned that they didn't think I would be here long at all. That made me smile.

James and Casey came in later that afternoon, and we went and checked out my daily schedule. I didn't have any classes until Monday. And I surprisingly had only a couple of classes a day, which would leave a lot of downtime for me. Still, there really wasn't any point for James and Casey to come during the day. I would be going to my classes alone, so it would be pointless for them to drive all the way to the other side of the city only to have to sit around and wait for me to finish each of my classes.

We hoped that I would still be able to go home in the evenings and weekends like I had before. We figured that James could pick me up once I had finished my classes and bring me back to sleep. I had just assumed that I would be allowed, but when I asked the nurse about it, she said that I would need to ask my doctor and he would have to decide. They usually didn't issue evening or weekend passes, unless that person was very close to being released.

I was scared. Being at home every evening and weekend had kept me sane. Being in my house, watching my own TV, hanging out with my family and friends, and sleeping in my own bed on weekends was the best part of my life right now. I couldn't imagine going back to being at the hospital day and night.

Unfortunately, my meeting with my new doctor was not until the next day, Friday. That meant I could not go home that evening, and I wouldn't know if I was going home for the weekend until the following day.

That evening, I just hung out with James and Casey, and once they left, I crawled into bed and read some magazines I had. My girlfriends had brought them for me months ago, but with me not being able to use my hands for so long, I had never even bothered trying to read them. By the time I could use my hands again, I always had someone around to talk to. For the first time in four months, I was alone. And although I thought it would be scary, it wasn't. I'd come such a long way from when I would have panic attacks anytime I was left alone. But now it actually felt really nice to have some me time.

I looked around my room. It was massive, and I had a huge bathroom with my own shower. It was three times the size of the one I had in my last room. This place was definitely designed for people in wheelchairs. I was really glad to be here, and I was definitely looking forward to my classes.

The next day, June 10, *Day 109*, James, Casey, and I spent the entire day in my room. I had no classes starting till Monday, and my doctor would be coming in to meet me sometime that day. The nurse couldn't predict when he would be coming to see me, so we were pretty much stuck in my room. I certainly didn't want to miss him as I wanted that weekend pass.

He didn't come till late afternoon. He first tested my strength and then told me he was expecting me to be a lot weaker. I had improved tremendously since I was assessed by their doctors six weeks before.

I asked him about the evening and weekend passes. He immediately told me that generally if someone is well enough to be at home on a pass, then they are well enough to be at home permanently. In his opinion, I was definitely not ready to be at home. Although I had improved drastically, I still had a long road to go.

My heart sank. I did not want to be stuck here all the time. But then he brought up another point. Although he didn't think I was ready for home passes, since I had been going home for over a month now, I had obviously found a way to function just fine. He didn't want to be the jerk to take my passes away when I had already been given them from someone else. I smiled. This meant I could still go home every evening and weekend.

I asked him how long he thought I would be here for. But he couldn't give me an answer. He told me that every Wednesday, the entire team who worked with me would meet and discuss my progress. They would generally come up with a release date right away. As things progressed, every Wednesday at their meetings, they would decide if that date needed to be changed or not.

Since I wouldn't be starting any physio classes till Monday, this Wednesday they would not have a meeting, seeing that I had only been there for a couple of days. They would not meet until the following Wednesday once they had all worked with me for a bit longer. That meant I would be here at least for thirteen days. This also meant that I would definitely be here past James' birthday, which was my original goal to be home by. The man who had had GBS before me had been here for three weeks, and I was really hoping it would be no longer than that for me too.

My doctor said that he wanted me to be fitted for AFO leg braces. The braces would immobilize my ankle, thereby making it safer when I walked. My ankles were definitely the weakest part of my body, and the braces would prevent my toes from dragging when I walked. He would set me up for a fitting next week. I was very worried how they would look. All I could picture in my head was Forest Gump and the leg braces he wore as a child.

My doctor also brought up how I had been through such a traumatic experience. He asked me if I had noticed any of my hair falling out. I had! He told me that it was quite common for hair to fall out about three months after severe emotional or physical stress. Now at least I knew there was an actual reason behind the increase in my hair shedding.

As soon as we were done with the doctor, we packed up my things and headed home for the weekend. I was so thankful to be able to continue going home.

That weekend was another weekend I did not want to miss out on. I was getting used to hearing about the different events I had missed, but now that I was getting out more often, I didn't want to miss a thing. My brother's girlfriend's daughter had her first birthday that Sunday, and I luckily would be able to attend.

We spent most of the weekend relaxing at home, and I continued to practice walking with the walker and going up and down the stairs. It was exhausting, and I was very slow, but it was getting a little easier each time I did it.

One surprising thing I learned was that I couldn't walk with flip-flops. The muscles in my feet weren't strong enough to keep the flip-flops on my feet. I had been wearing slip-on runners since I had started wearing shoes again, and this meant that I would most likely be wearing them all summer.

On Sunday, we went to the birthday party. My friends were happy to see me out and about once again. I was, too. Casey had always loved being around the nurses and doctors in the hospital, but it was then that I noticed just how much she loved being around people in general, especially other kids. She lit up whenever she was around a large group of people. She would just stare and watch every single person. It was like she was studying them. She was so attentive to everything going on around her. She was almost five months old, and her personality was really starting to shine through.

There was a kiddie pool set up for the kids, and my mom put Casey in it. This was the first time she had ever been in a pool. And she loved it. I was disappointed that I couldn't be the one to hold her in the pool, but I was so happy I was able to be here to see her in it for the first time. I really felt like I was a part of her life now. I absolutely loved watching her grow.

Monday, June 13, *Day 112*, was my first day by myself at the hospital. Breakfast was brought into my room, and I had my first class, which was physiotherapy shortly after. I wasn't sure where to go, so I had a porter bring me down.

My physiotherapist spent most of the class assessing me, in order to figure out where I was and what we needed to work on. After she was done, she commented that she really didn't think that I would be here long. That made me extremely happy.

Once I was done, the porter brought me back to my room. I didn't have any classes until after lunchtime, which was over an hour away. My mom had left me her laptop, so I went on the Internet for that hour. The door to my room was open, and the patient across from me wheeled by and said, "Hello," then mentioned that if I wanted to get out of my room, I could certainly use my laptop in the cafeteria, or if it was nice out, then outside. That's what he always did. I appreciated the suggestion, but I was still nervous about wheeling myself around. I hadn't wheeled around on my own for any long period of time, so I was scared that I wouldn't be able to do it. For the time being, I just wanted to stay in my room.

The nurse brought my lunch to my room, and later, I had my next class, which was occupational therapy. Their job was to help me to improve my basic motor functions as well as to help me to get back to everyday activities.

Just like the physiotherapists, they were surprised to see how much farther I was in my recovery. They were usually the ones that helped patients learn how to transfer, which I had already mastered. But there were still a few things she was able to help me with. One thing was a way for me to put on my socks and shoes. James, my mom, or my nurses were still doing that for me. She showed me how to lie in bed and lean over to put them on, which was actually possible compared to bending over in my chair, which was not.

The second thing she showed me was how to transfer onto a toilet seat raiser, instead of the commode. Instead of a commode chair that went over the toilet, the raiser fit right on top of the seat. There were two bars along the sides of it that I could use to push up to a standing position. By using this, I was using my arms way more. This helped strengthen them so that eventually I would be able to push myself up on my own without the bars. Once I knew I was comfortable using it at the hospital, we brought back the commode from home and exchanged it for the seat.

When she was done with the assessment, she told me that she would be putting me into a hand class, which would help me with my fine motor skills, as well as stretch and further strengthen my upper body. My upper body was definitely stronger than my lower body, but I knew that it still needed a lot of work.

After the class, I decided to attempt to wheel myself back to my room. It was pretty far away and on a whole other floor.

It wasn't as hard as I thought it would be, and I made it back fine, but I moved pretty slowly. As I wheeled by, one of the other patients told me it would get easier. I must have been really slow!

I was all done for the day, so I had James pick me up, and we headed home. We had dinner and watched some TV and then, a few hours later, James brought me back to the hospital.

I crawled into bed, read a magazine, went on Facebook, and then went to sleep. This would be my routine for quite some time.

The following day, I started working out in physiotherapy. They worked my legs by having me stand in the parallel bars for support and then do squats. I couldn't believe my balance. I could not stand there without at least having one hand on the bar. When she asked me to try walking without holding on, I just couldn't do it.

We also practiced walking with the walker, and we walked around the unit. I was able to walk around twice, and when we were done for the day, I wasn't tired one bit. I was confident that I could keep going if I wanted.

Later that day, I was fitted for the braces. I was shown what they would look like, and I was happy to see that they were just a brace that fit to the back of your leg and strapped on. They were made of plastic and could fit under my pants just fine. I could also pick the pattern I wanted, and I picked the leopard print.

The following day, I started another new class, where we would meet with the other patients on our ward and talk about the different problems we were each facing. When everyone around the room talked about what had brought each of them there, I was surprised. I couldn't believe how many people had serious spinal cord issues, and many of them weren't sure if they would ever walk again. I couldn't help but feel lucky.

We got to one man in the circle, and he started talking about his Guillain-Barré syndrome. I couldn't believe it! Someone else was here with what I had! He was older, probably in his forties and was in a motorized wheelchair. As he talked, I learned that his recovery was taking a long time, a lot longer than mine. He had been diagnosed with GBS in January and was nowhere near where I was.

That afternoon, I started my hand class in which I worked on my upper body. I then worked on my fine motor skills by doing things like using a tiny screwdriver to take out these tiny screws and then picking up each of the screws and screwing them into tiny little holes. This drove me crazy. I was still pretty shaky, and I dropped them over and over again. But I could certainly see that with practice it would get easier.

They tested my coordination, but thankfully, it was pretty much back to normal. I had no problem grabbing safety pins and placing them in a jar over and over again. I had mastered this back in the other hospital, with the cones.

That night, back at home, James and I watched hockey. The Stanley Cup was on. I had gotten quite used to watching hockey in both my rooms back at the other hospital. Vancouver was playing against Boston. We were cheering for Vancouver, the last Canadian team standing, but unfortunately they lost.

I went back to the hospital afterward, and some of the patients on my ward were sitting in the TV area, talking about the Stanley Cup game. I wheeled up and talked about it with them for a few minutes, then went back to my room.

I relaxed in my bed, once again reading through the magazines and checking my Facebook. I couldn't believe that tomorrow would mark the end of a week in this place. I was starting to get lonely. I missed my husband and my baby girl greatly. I was used to being with them every day, and it broke my heart that I wasn't home with them. I just wanted to go home.

One thing that I noticed while I lay in my bed was just how sore my hips were. My hip bones were just aching, which I assumed was from all the walking I was now doing.

At my next physio class, as I waited for my therapist to be done with another patient, I got to talking to a man also waiting for his therapist. He was probably in his sixties. I asked him why he was here, and why he was in a wheelchair. He said that it was because of Guillain-Barré syndrome. I couldn't believe I was meeting yet another person with GBS. We exchanged stories; his wasn't as severe as mine as he was never in the ICU, but his recovery was taking longer. This was most likely due to his age as well. He had been diagnosed around the same time as me but had yet to even try walking.

My mom came to visit that day, and since she was joining me for lunch, we decided to eat in the cafeteria. I had yet to eat in there; I was still eating lunch in my own room.

The patient from across the hall said hi and told me that it was nice to see me out of my room. He told me I should come downstairs with everyone on their breaks to have a smoke. When I told him I didn't smoke, he told me I could always come down for the company. Sitting in my room must be getting quite boring. He was right. I was getting pretty lonely all by myself.

Later that evening, instead of going home, my mom and I went shopping. James' birthday, which was also falling on Father's Day, was coming up this weekend, and I needed to get him something for both. I settled on clothes for his birthday and a fancy pulsating shower head for Father's Day. I knew he had always wanted one, and now that he was a full-time dad, I felt it was appropriate to give him something for the home.

June 17, *Day 116*, after my physio class, I decided to venture outside. There were quite a few people out there, everyone in wheelchairs. Almost everyone was smoking, but there were a few, like me, that had just gone out for the company. Someone asked me what I was in there for, and everyone laughed. It sounded like we were talking about jail, like we had each done something wrong to end up there. When I told them what I had, no one had heard of it, and it was hard to explain in a few sentences.

I learned that the patient across the hall from me had something very rare happen to the nerves in his spine. They had intertwined, which basically paralyzed him from the waist down. He would most likely never walk again. Another patient I met, a girl, who was a few years older than me, had fallen off a ledge and broken her back. She would definitely never walk again. Hearing them say this really broke my heart.

That afternoon was a blast. It felt great to be meeting and talking with other people. It was nice to talk to people that were also dealing with such traumatic events in their lives. It's not that my family wasn't supportive; they were unbelievable, but to be able to talk with people who had been through something like me was very therapeutic.

When I left to go back upstairs, they all told me they would see me later that night, or sometime that weekend. But I wouldn't, as it was Friday, and I was going home for another weekend pass. When I told them that, they were completely surprised. Not many people got weekend passes here. They were obviously quite envious of me, and I felt extremely grateful that I was able to go home and be with my family.

That night, James had his birthday party at our house. My girlfriend from out of town was up, and a lot of our friends that we hadn't seen in a while came out for it. It felt so normal being at home. Although slow, I was a pro at the stairs and did them comfortably by myself all the time now. I didn't even bring my wheelchair in from James' truck and got around my house using my walker instead. I even had the guts to take a few steps from my walker to the table. I amazed everyone, especially myself, by not falling. I was so wobbly! I felt like a baby taking her first steps.

On Saturday, my girlfriends wanted to go see *Bridesmaids*, a new movie that was playing. I knew that there were spots for people in wheelchairs to sit, so I could actually go with them to see it.

When we got to the theatre, we were shocked to see how busy it was. The lineup was massive, and we were worried we wouldn't make it on time. Luckily, a staff member saw me in my wheelchair and called us up to the front of the line. I was very appreciative.

Unfortunately, the movie we wanted to see was sold out. The woman said that there might be a few random seats, but it was highly unlikely there would be any together. We decided to take a look as we thought that maybe the spot beside the wheelchair area would be open, but it wasn't.

We went back to my place, and along with my brother and James, we watched a movie and then played some board games. Playing board games proved to be even better than going to the movies. The game we played was hilarious, and I laughed harder than I had laughed in a really long time. It felt like my normal life again.

Sunday was James' actual birthday and his first father's day. It was also eight years ago that day that we had started dating. It was unbelievable to think about what we had gone through this past year together.

Casey was learning to use her voice and was really starting to babble that day. She was also starting to laugh at everything. I still couldn't pick her up on my own, but we found a way that she could be with me as I walked around the house. We set her Bumbo chair onto the seat of my walker and then James placed her in it. I could now walk around the house with her sitting right on my walker! I loved being a part of her life.

When we got back to the hospital after the weekend was over, I saw some of the people I had met on Friday sitting outside. I usually just had James drop me off at the front doors and went up to my room on my own, but I had him drive me over to where everyone was sitting. It was close to nine o'clock, and I wanted to be in bed by ten, so I was nice and rested for physio the next day. I figured I would chat for a bit and then head off to bed.

Before I knew it, it was almost midnight, and we were heading back in before they locked the doors for the night.

I had met quite a few different people that night, and it was nice to get to know some of the other patients being rehabilitated there.

I met a young guy from up north who had broken his back in a sledding accident. I thought he meant sledding as in snowmobiling, but he actually meant sledding as in tobogganing. He would never walk again. I couldn't believe that something so innocent could cause so much damage.

I met another young guy that had been jumped on his walk to a 7-Eleven store. He was beaten up so badly that he suffered severe brain damage, so he couldn't even talk. He communicated with a tiny computer that spoke for him when he typed. He would be in a wheelchair for the rest of his life.

Another man I met, had come to the hospital with symptoms similar to mine—weakness and paralysis. It wasn't GBS, though; it was very likely multiple sclerosis (MS), and it was possible that he would not walk again either.

When I went to bed that night, I couldn't help but feel extremely lucky. The majority of the people I met here would never walk again. Their lives were changed forever. They would have to learn how to function in everyday life, in wheelchairs, for the rest of their lives. Yes, my journey so far had been extremely challenging, and I still had a long way to go. But one day, I would be out of my wheelchair. It would take time, but my life would eventually return to normal, and I would walk again. I couldn't think of too many diseases that allowed for that. I really started to realize that things could have been way worse, and I was actually grateful that all I had was Guillain-Barré syndrome.

Monday, June 20, *Day 119*, I got my AFO braces for my legs. They were stiff and awkward, but they definitely made my legs feel sturdier when I tried walking with them in physiotherapy. And the leopard print looked pretty cool.

My body was definitely recovering, and everything continued to get better and easier every day. The week before, I couldn't stand on my own without holding onto something. This week, I could. Last week, I couldn't lift my arms back far enough to put my hair up. This week, I finally could! I was now able to write with a pen, and in my hand class, I could lift more than I could when I had started just a week before. I could even do a full flight of stairs without feeling tired at all.

And then came the best news. My physiotherapist was thrilled to tell me that I was ready to start walking with the walker, all the time. I had been using it around my house and in physio, but I hadn't used it outside of either yet. But the more I actually walked, the longer I would be able to go. So from now on, I would get around everywhere using my walker. This was such a huge step! I was no longer in a wheelchair!

Since I no longer needed to practice with the walker, I now spent my time in physio practicing with a cane. My PT held onto the transfer belt around my waist as I walked. I was so wobbly and didn't have much balance, but with my PT holding on, I could do it. I was nowhere near being able to walk with a cane outside of physio, but I knew that the more I practiced, the easier it would get.

Because I wasn't able to squat, I couldn't physically pick up Casey, so my physiotherapists taught me how to get right down onto the floor. That way, I could at least play with her on the floor. I couldn't imagine how on earth I was going to get from my walker onto the floor. I could walk, but I could barely squat down a few inches before my ankles would start to shake and give out on me.

I was shown how to get onto the floor, with the help from my walker, by using it to lean on to bend down onto one knee. Being on one of my knees took the pressure off my ankles, which gave me enough strength to get down onto the other knee. Once I was on all fours, I would just move and wiggle my body around into a sitting position. To get back up was exactly the same, backward. I would get onto all fours and then, with the help from my walker, pull myself up on one leg. Then I could easily just push myself up onto the other leg. Although it was a little painful on my ankles, it was actually quite easy. And I was really happy

I would be able to get down onto the ground to play with my baby girl. My physiotherapy was helping me in such a huge way.

Between physio sessions, about three to four times a day, I would sit outside with all the smokers, talking and laughing. There were always quite a few people outside, but I found myself spending most of my time with the same three people—two of the older guys, the one who likely had MS and the other that had a rare disorder in his nerves, and the girl who had been paralyzed from falling off a balcony. These three were the most outgoing of the group and absolutely hilarious! Everything that came out of their mouths was so funny, and we had such a great time laughing all day long. When I look back on my journey with GBS, some of my most favorite memories were with these three patients. They constantly made me smile and laugh, and we had such a great time together.

Not only did these three people make me laugh, they also amazed me. The three of them, who would likely never walk again, were the most positive and cheerful people there. I thought it was amazing that even though they would likely be in wheelchairs forever, they didn't let it ruin their lives. They didn't let it bring them down, and they certainly didn't let it stop their personalities from shining through. They were still the same outgoing, happy, and funny people I'm sure they were before their accidents.

When I started using my walker outside, instead of my wheelchair, all the other patients were amazed. Although we had talked about my disorder, most people just assumed that I would not walk again, like the majority of the patients on my ward. When I told them that I would likely recover completely, I could see just how happy they were for me. And this really inspired me. That even though their lives would never be the same, they could still share in my joy.

I was so close to being able to walk all on my own again; I was reaching my goals every single day, and I had so much to be thankful for. If they could be this happy and positive, then I knew I had more than enough reasons to be happy and positive as well.

Every evening, I was still going home with James and Casey for dinner, and every night I would return to the hospital. We started calling our group that hung outside "The Flock," and I would have James drop me off near "The Flock," so I could spend a few hours with them until I went to bed.

On Wednesday, June 22, *Day 121*, exactly four months of being in a hospital, my doctor came in to talk to me about my discharge date from the hospital. He first started by telling me that although I had improved drastically, I still had a long way to go. And if it weren't for my husband being at home to take care of me, he probably wouldn't even be letting me go home on weekends. But in view of the fact that James was at home all the time and that he wasn't working and wouldn't be going back to work till October, he felt that I was almost ready to go home. If James was still working and not able to take care of me, he would be keeping me for at least another three weeks. Instead, my release date would be the following Tuesday.

That meant that in only six days I would be going home for good! I almost couldn't believe it. I was unbelievably excited. I was certainly enjoying my time here; the company was fantastic, and the therapy was helping immensely. But to be back home with my husband and daughter was all that I really wanted. And I couldn't believe that in less than a week, I would be back with my family again. I would be back to sleeping in my own bed every single night. And back to my normal life every single day. Back to being me. I could not wait.

The following evening, a friend of ours had a BBQ, and once I had done my physio for the day, we headed over there. It was the first time I was using my walker outside of the house or the hospital. I always wore my AFO braces when I practiced walking, but on this particular day, it was extremely hot outside, and the plastic on my legs made it even worse. I chose not to wear them.

When we got to our friend's place, as usual, everyone was happy to see how much I had improved since the last time they had seen me.

This was the first time they had seen me without my wheelchair, and I knew they were proud of me.

I was thrilled to announce to my friends that I would be going home in less than a week. Everyone was extremely excited for me, but their excitement quickly transferred over to the hosts of the BBQ, who announced their pregnancy! It was such a joyous evening, and I was so happy that I was able to be there and be a part of the celebration. I couldn't wait to have my life back and to start being a part of everyone's lives again.

The last few days of the week went by very quickly. Since I was going home Tuesday, and would spend Monday packing up, all my physiotherapy sessions would be finished by the end of the week. I was assessed by each of my physiotherapists one last time, so they could see just how much I had improved. And it was really amazing to see how much I had changed in just a few short weeks.

The most obvious change was in my walking; I had come in a wheelchair and I would leave using a walker. But it definitely wasn't the only thing that I had improved on. Less than two weeks ago, I was struggling to wheel myself around the hallways. Now I was a pro; I wheeled myself around with no problems, very quickly. When I first arrived, James was transferring me in and out of my wheelchair into the truck. Now I could get in and out of his truck all on my own. My body was so much stronger now, and I couldn't have been more thrilled.

My weekend at home was my last weekend pass. The next time I was home would be for good. We spent the weekend relaxing at home, and things couldn't have been better. I was so close to getting my life back. And when I went back to the hospital on Sunday night, although I thought it would be hard, it wasn't. I was still looking forward to saying good-bye to all the amazing people I had met.

On Monday morning, June 27, *Day 126*, my doctor came in to talk to me. Although I wasn't supposed to leave until Tuesday morning, I was finished with my physio, and the patient that would be taking my room was ready to be transferred. This meant I could go home today. Once I was finished packing, I could leave.

When I called both James and my mom to tell them the good news, neither of them could control their happiness. Even though it was only one day early, they still weren't expecting it, and they were overcome with joy.

Casey had just gone down for a nap at the time I called James, so instead of having him wake her up, my mom came to the hospital to bring me home. As I finished packing up my room, I looked around, knowing that this would be the last time I would be in this hospital room. And I couldn't have been happier. I said my good-byes to everyone and made my way outside.

Once my mom arrived, she took a few pictures of me in front of the hospital and then we got in her van and headed home. I had made the trip from the hospital to my house a million times, but this time was different. I knew I would never be returning to sleep at this hospital again.

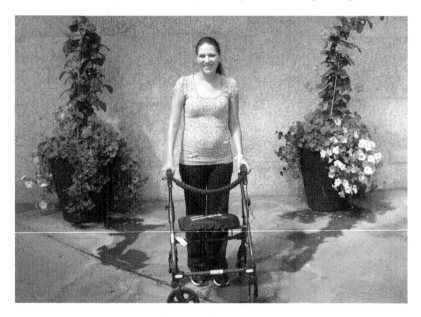

Leaving the Rehabilitation Hospital after a total of 126 days in the hospital

When I got home, James and Casey came outside. We put Casey in her Bumbo chair on my walker, and I walked into my house. It truly was a magical experience. After spending 126 days in the hospital, I was home. I was ready to start my life again with my family. I couldn't wait to pick things back up right where I had left them four months before.

My first night home was fantastic. It almost didn't feel real! I was so used to being at the hospital all the time that it felt strange when I didn't have to go back at the end of the day. I had gotten so used to being there all the time. That place had been my home for three weeks, and I had made some great friends. But as much as I had enjoyed my last few weeks there, I knew I could never be happier than I was now.

The following day, after my first official day at home, James, Casey, and I went out for an early dinner to celebrate. I used my walker to walk and left the wheelchair at home.

It felt really strange being around regular people with my walker. Although I was used to walking with it, I had only been around friends or at the hospital and hadn't really been seen out in public with it. I knew that I looked different, but I certainly didn't like to feel different. I knew that people were looking at me, probably wondering what on earth I had that would require me to use a walker at my age.

The waitress had to seat us at a certain table, so there was room for me to put my walker, and I felt uncomfortable that they had to make special arrangements for me. But seeing that I had no idea when I would be able to walk on my own, I knew that I had no choice but to accept it.

When we were done eating, I asked James if he wanted to go shopping. I hadn't shopped in months and really wanted to get some new clothes. I didn't feel like me. I was still really hot all the time; therefore, I didn't have the energy to straighten my hair, and when I looked in the mirror, I still didn't see me. I figured some retail therapy could help me feel better about myself.

But James wasn't in the mood to go shopping; he really just wanted to get home and relax. I was disappointed, but I knew how much work it was to take care of Casey and me. He was doing so much for us already, and I didn't want to push him. Besides, I knew there were many more days that we could go shopping.

When we pulled into the garage, as I walked with my walker into the backyard, I noticed my back door was open. I had to lift my walker over the lip of the door frame, and as I lifted, I then noticed my mom's dogs staring out from inside the house. I thought to myself, "Oh, my mom must have stopped by to say hi." Once I had my walker placed on the pavement for me to walk, all of a sudden, I heard "Surprise!" I looked to my right, and there stood all of my closest friends and family with a huge banner that read, "Welcome Home!"

I couldn't believe it! That's why James didn't want to go shopping! I was shocked; I had absolutely no idea that my husband had been planning this surprise for me.

We spent the next few hours eating, hanging out, and opening welcome-home gifts. It was so nice to be home for good. I had so many amazing people in my life.

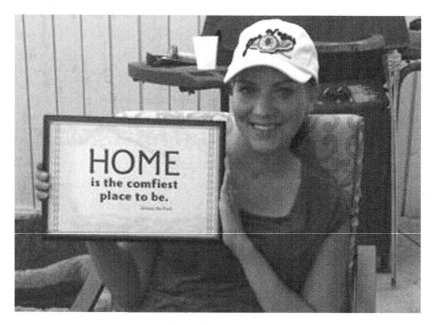

Home Sweet Home

July

My life was slowly getting back to normal. I was back to being a mother and a wife and no longer just a hospital patient. My life no longer revolved around my disability. I certainly was still limited because of it, but it no longer consumed my entire day.

I loved being able to get out and about, but I quickly learned that I didn't have the energy that I used to have. After getting out of the house to run errands with James for two straight days, I was exhausted and couldn't get off my couch. Even getting up to get something was too tiring, so James had to do most things for me. I could go up and down the stairs without any problems, but when I was done, I was out of breath and had to lie down. I eventually learned only to go upstairs once or twice a day, as the very thought of going up them overwhelmed me.

I felt really guilty. It was summer, and gorgeous outside, but I just didn't have the energy to get up and out of the house as often as I would have liked. I knew James was bored, and I knew he didn't want to sit around watching movies all day long, but he did, for me, for several straight days. I had such a great husband.

As I went through my days, I figured out what I could do and what I couldn't do. I had come a long way from the days that I could barely hold a pen, or even push a button on a remote control, but I certainly wasn't back to normal. I was limited to my walker, so I couldn't help with the cooking or any chores. I couldn't even open baby bottles, so I had to have James open them whenever we had to feed Casey. James pretty much did everything around the house.

Although my leg muscles were getting stronger every day, I still couldn't squat at all. My legs were strong enough to hold me up, but they still weren't strong enough for me to bend down at all. I couldn't bend down to pick up Casey, so James carried her everywhere. I couldn't even bend down to put my shoes on, so the majority of the time I wore slip-on flats.

I was also a lot more tired than usual and slept more than ten hours a night, as well as napping during the day. I was quite amazed at how much energy it took to walk.

My favorite part of being home was being a mom again. I loved holding Casey in my arms and just staring into her eyes. I loved getting to feed and change her all the time, instead of just some of the time. I loved her so much.

Things weren't going exactly the way I had pictured them, though. Whenever Casey would cry, I just couldn't get her to stop. I would cuddle and kiss her and try to calm her down, but it wouldn't work. James would come up and grab her, and she instantly would stop crying. At first, I thought I was doing something wrong, but then I realized what it was. She didn't know me. I mean, yes, she knew me as a person, but she didn't know me as her parent. I hadn't been the one who had fed her, changed her, burped her, and rocked her every single day for the last four months. I hadn't been the one that had fixed things for her whenever she cried. That was James, and that's who she wanted.

Not only that, but I wasn't on top of things the way James was. Casey would cry, and I wouldn't know why, and James would say, "Oh, she's hungry, that's why," or "she needs to be changed." He was used to taking care of a baby; I wasn't. I felt guilty that I didn't know her the way a mother should know her baby.

I would try and try to get Casey to laugh, but I could only ever manage to get a smile out of her. James would do one small thing, and she would giggle hysterically for ten minutes straight. I was extremely jealous of the relationship my husband had with my daughter, and I choked back tears every time she wanted her daddy instead of me.

Now that I was home, James and I started making a plan on what to do with the money that was raised for us at the fundraiser. The first thing we wanted to do was pay off all of our debt. James was on employment insurance (EI), and I was on disability, which was a significant amount less than our usual monthly income. James would need to be my caregiver, as well as Casey's, for a while, and would not be going back to work till October. And neither of us knew when I would be going back to work. We didn't want to stress about money, and we knew that by paying off all the debt we had, we would have one less thing to worry about down the road.

We put over two-thirds of the money into a savings account; some of it would help pay our bills every month until we were both working again, and the rest would be saved for the future. We also put some money into our retirement fund, and some went into Casey's education fund. Neither James' nor my parents had a lot of money growing up, and with this extra money we would be able to do some of the things for Casey that I'm sure our parents wished they could have done for us.

I couldn't have been more grateful for what my friends had done for us. This whole ordeal was the most stressful and challenging thing I had ever faced in my life, and knowing that I didn't have to stress over paying our bills was such a huge relief. Knowing that my daughter would be taken care of not only now but also in the future was also very comforting.

If it hadn't been for the fundraiser, we would have gone tens of thousands of dollars into debt, struggling to pay our bills. If it hadn't been for all the amazing donations, we would not have been able to keep up.

As the weeks went by, and as I gained more balance and strength in my legs, I started walking with Casey's stroller instead of my walker whenever we left the house. It provided me with the same amount of stability, and this way I didn't look so out of place. I was still extremely slow, but I knew that it was a step in the right direction.

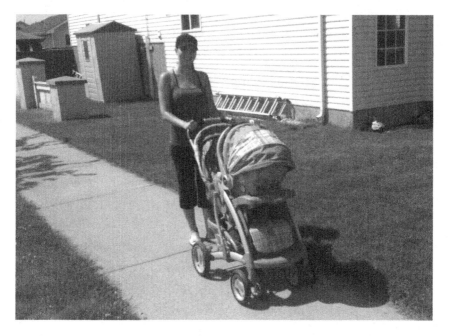

Practicing walking with Casey's stroller

One night, James and I got a babysitter, and we joined my brother and his girlfriend to go see a movie. I brought my wheelchair instead of my walker, so that I would be able to sit in that in the handicapped section of the theater.

But when we got there, once again it was extremely busy, and there weren't enough seats beside where the wheelchair would go. There were some seats a few rows below. I figured I had to start somewhere. I decided to put my wheelchair in the designated spot, and with help from James, I would walk down and over to the available seats.

I knew that people were staring at me as I struggled to get up from my chair, and while holding onto James, I hobbled my way down the steps and over to our seats. I plopped down into my seat. The chair was extremely low, and I knew it would be even harder for me to get out of it.

Once the movie was over, I had to have James lift me to a standing position as I just didn't have the strength in my arms and legs to push myself to stand. Then by holding onto James and the nearby seats, I slowly made my way back to my wheelchair.

I was extremely proud of myself. I had to hold onto James to walk, but I knew that it wouldn't be long before I would be walking all on my own. I made the decision to abandon my walker and start using the cane from now on.

Using the cane was a lot more difficult, and it made my walking even slower than I already was. Keeping my balance was a lot harder with having only one hand on something instead of both, and without the help from the wheels on the walker, I walked very, very slowly.

My girlfriend, who had gotten the job on the cruise ship, was finally going to the Caribbean to work by the end of the month. Her contract was for six months, and I couldn't believe that I wouldn't see her for that long. She decided to have a small get-together at her parents' cabin, about an hour and a half away, for a camping trip before she left. At first, we didn't think we were going to go; I didn't think I was up for it, but after thinking about it some more, I changed my mind. I didn't want my disability holding me back from living my life.

We brought Casey to Grandma and Grandpa's and headed out there on Saturday, July 16. I brought just my cane. We got to the campsite and had some drinks around the campfire. It was a really sunny day, and everyone decided that they wanted to head for the beach. I couldn't wear flip-flops, so I wore a pair of water shoes. The few drinks I had hit me harder than normal, and the liquid courage told me that I didn't need to bring my cane. I figured I would just walk holding onto someone.

When we got to the beach, one of my girlfriends held my hand as we walked toward the water. I had walked with help from James a few times and figured I would be fine as long as I had someone to hold onto. But as soon as we got onto the sand, I realized I was in over my head. The sand was completely different than concrete, and it was a lot harder to keep my balance on the uneven ground. I was barely able to stand, so my girlfriend grabbed onto both my hands and walked in front of me, as I slowly walked.

We threw our air mattresses into the lake and jumped on them to float. It wasn't as warm out on the lake, but we hoped that the sunshine would still give us a tan. I remember jumping into the lake and then trying to get back up onto the mattress, but I couldn't. I didn't have the strength in my body to hoist myself back up onto the mattress. James had to pull me up. I was definitely figuring out what my body was capable of doing and what it wasn't.

The rest of the camping trip went smoothly, and after having some good laughs with great friends, we headed back home.

My friends and family had always been very important to me, but if I learned anything from this whole experience, it was just how amazing they truly were by the way they had been there with me during this time. I knew that not only did I need to spend more time with the people I loved, but also I needed to start living my life to the fullest. When I really wanted to do something, instead of putting it off, I needed to just do it. No one is ever promised tomorrow, so I needed to do the things I wanted to do today.

It was only a few days after the camping trip that we packed up the car, Casey, and the dogs and headed out to Golden, BC. My cousin had moved there a few weeks earlier, and I couldn't wait to see him in his new place.

My cousin and I are extremely close; he is more like a brother to me. He was living over twenty hours away when I was in the hospital, but he had managed to get some time off work to visit me. Shortly after he had returned home, he himself had some health problems that had landed him in the hospital. They weren't as serious as mine, but after the year we both had had, we really wanted to spend some time together. And now that he was only about five hours away, the first weekend that we both had free, we jumped at the chance to get together.

I had learned my lesson when camping that I was nowhere near ready to walk without my cane. So I was sure to bring it everywhere I went. My cousin had last seen me at my very worst, when I was still completely paralyzed in my hospital bed. So when he saw me physically walking, I know it made him very happy.

We expected the weather to be gorgeous, but unfortunately, it was cloudy and rainy the whole weekend. We had planned to spend most of our time outside but we were at a loss of what to do in this crappy weather. On the first day, we decided to drive down to Radium Hot Springs. It was only an hour away, but the weather said it was sunny there.

I chose to wear my bikini. I was extremely self-conscious of the scar on my neck, but I wasn't as bothered by the scar on my stomach anymore. When we walked into the pool, I knew that people were staring at us. My cousin felt it too, and he told me that he wondered what they thought when they saw me. It definitely was not every day that you saw someone my age walking with a cane, with a massive scar down their torso.

Although I knew I stood out, I didn't let it get in the way of enjoying our day. It was Casey's first time in the mountains, her first time swimming, and I wanted this to be fun time for everyone. Even when it started raining and then hailing, I didn't let it ruin things. James held Casey close to his body and shielded her head with his hands as the hail came down on us. A few people started leaving, but I wanted to wait it out, hoping that it would be over soon. And I was right. A few minutes later, the sun came out again. I couldn't help but laugh; Casey was such a trooper and didn't seem bothered by the storm one bit. She just loved being in the water.

The following day, it was pouring, but we headed out to Field, about half an hour away. My cousin had told us that there was a huge waterfall out there, and it was a beautiful view. And once we got there, he was right; it was just gorgeous. We were parked quite far away, so James and my cousin took a short hike to get a better view. I wanted to go, but I knew that there was no way I could physically walk on a trail. I knew my ankles were just not strong enough for any major walking yet, so I stayed in the car with Casey.

Just before we left, when we went to change Casey, we realized that we had forgotten the diaper bag. We were in the middle of the mountains, and of course Casey had leaked through her diaper and through her pants. We headed out to a gas station on the side of the road, and James ran in hopes of finding diapers and wipes, but they didn't have either. My cousin and I laughed so hard when James came back to the car with toilet paper and wet naps. We cleaned Casey up as best we could and then wrapped her in a receiving blanket until we were home. It definitely wasn't the best thing we did as parents, but when I look back on it, I can't help but laugh.

And although the weather never did let up for the rest of our trip, we made the best of it and had a really great time that weekend.

Once we were home from our trip, I e-mailed my respiratory therapist, the one that had offered us his home in Phoenix. Getting away for the weekend with James and Casey had been so nice, but what I really wanted was to go somewhere where I could just lie in the sun all day. My body couldn't handle too much excursion, so I knew that lying by the pool would be just what I needed.

We e-mailed back and forth, discussing possible dates for us to go, and we came up with the end of September. That would still give me two months to improve on my walking. Our wedding anniversary was also September 19, so we could celebrate it there. I was astonished when he wrote back to say that the place was completely free in September and October, so we were welcome to stay as long as we wanted.

I had initially thought we could go for two weeks, but James convinced me to go for three weeks. He reminded me of what I had gone through during these past months and told me that I deserved to have a nice, long vacation. He wanted us both to forget this entire nightmare and spend time as a family in paradise. Not only that, but it really wouldn't cost us more to stay longer. We didn't have to pay for accommodation, so an extra week would only cost us groceries, which we would be paying for at home anyway. If we left just before our anniversary and stayed for three weeks, then James would go back to work when we got back. It did sound like the perfect end to this whole ordeal.

So it was settled. We would go for three weeks to Phoenix in September. He had also mentioned in his e-mail that we were welcome to bring other guests, since the home was a four-bedroom house. Originally, we had hoped that either my brother and his girlfriend or my mom and stepfather could join us, but the timing just didn't work for everyone. In the end, it was just my mom who decided to come for a week.

As usual, I continued to amaze myself with my recovery. I found myself needing to use the cane less and less. I no longer used it in the house at all; I simply ran my fingers along the walls to keep my balance. When we were out, I either used the stroller or a shopping cart to help me walk. The wheelchair and walker were now sitting in the garage collecting dust. The only thing I still used was the shower seat. I didn't quite have the balance to stand on my own for that long. I couldn't even put my pants on without having to lean against my bed to lift each leg. But I knew I would eventually be able to do it all. I was improving all the time.

Before I knew it, my best friend was leaving for her new job on the cruise ship. I was so happy for her; I knew this was her dream job come true, but I was extremely sad to see her go. She and I never went for more than a few days without talking, and I knew that we wouldn't get to talk very often at all. The hardest part would be going six whole months before seeing her again. We drove her to the airport and said our good-byes.

I was so glad that I was well enough to see her fulfill her dream. She had literally gotten the job the day that I was diagnosed with Guillain-Barré syndrome, but it had taken months to get her work visa in order. And although I knew the wait had been very hard for her, secretly I couldn't have been happier. That meant that she was there for me while I dealt with the most terrifying experience of my life. I couldn't imagine if she had left when I was at my worst.

Just before she left, CTV News contacted her regarding my recovery. They wanted to do a follow-up story on me, and she had provided me with the reporter's phone number. When I called them, we arranged a date for them to interview us.

It was only a few days later, on July 26, that they came, and already I was better than I had been just days before. When they interviewed me, they had me walk up the stairs into Casey's room to show just how much I had improved. I didn't even use the walls to walk. I was pretty wobbly and struggled to keep my balance, but I wanted to show the world that I was finally much better.

The follow-up story aired that evening, and we couldn't have been happier with the way they did it. CTV news had wanted to show their viewers what had happened to me, and we were all glad to show a happy ending to our story.

My first month back at home was wonderful, and I couldn't have been more grateful to be back with my family. I had never realized just how amazing my life really was until this happened, and it definitely made me appreciate everything so much more.

My ESBL bladder infection did go away eventually, and my doctors took me off the antidepressant medication. Now all I was on was the medication for the nerve pain.

Casey was another month older, now six months old. She was starting to sit up on her own. She got her first two teeth, and she started eating solids all within days of each other. Being home to witness all this was such a gift. To me, even being able to change my daughter's diaper was a blessing. It's something most people take for granted. But I truly appreciated it. It was very fulfilling to know that, at one point, I was not even strong enough to hold a diaper in my hand, but now I could change her all on my own.

Squatting was still very hard, but I was learning how to hold on to things as I bent down to pick them up. I remember that every time I saw someone squat, it would make me cringe, knowing the amount of pain it would cause in my ankles. I was, however, strong enough to push myself up from a sitting position, so I no longer used the toilet seat raiser anymore. My legs were strong enough to push my legs on the stairs, so I could now use alternate legs, rather than going up them one step at a time.

I still didn't feel like myself, though, and it was hard to explain that to people. I still felt hotter than the average person; I rarely wore a sweater, I slept without blankets, and I couldn't blow-dry or straighten my hair without feeling like I was going to faint. On top of my hair constantly being a wavy mess, it was falling out even more now. My hair was so much thinner than usual, and I just didn't see me when I looked in the mirror.

The scar on my neck was still very noticeable, but I figured out that I could use cover up to hide it a teeny bit. I knew I had no reason to cover it up; I had no reason to be embarrassed over it, but I hated it and was extremely self-conscious about it.

Everything I had read told me that my voice would get stronger and stronger and return to normal, but it wasn't. It was still extremely low and hoarse, and I was constantly asked if I had a cold. I came to the conclusion that my vocal cords must have been damaged by the breathing tube, and that was why it was not getting stronger. I was also extremely self-conscious over it.

The hypersensitivity in my feet was actually getting worse. My feet had been completely numb for months, but now that the nerves were regenerating in my feet, they constantly hurt. Stepping on a tiny pebble felt like I was stepping on shards of glass. When my dogs would step on my feet, I would scream in pain. And at the end of the day, my feet would ache and throb like I had walked miles and miles on them in bare feet.

Despite everything that still hadn't returned to normal yet, I was still very happy. I was grateful for my life and all the amazing things in it.

By the end of July, after a long five months, I reached my ultimate goal. I could officially say that I was walking again, by myself! I no longer used the cane anymore at all. It took a lot of concentration to keep my balance; my legs got sore very quickly, and I was extremely slow, but I was walking on my own again, and that's all that mattered.

August

Although I was determined not to use my cane anymore, I found I was a lot faster when I walked with Casey's stroller. We had gone to a football game one evening, without Casey, and I struggled to keep up with everyone else. My legs were aching so badly by the time we got home that for most of my trips outside our home, I continued to use the stroller to help me walk.

On August Long Weekend, we headed out to Slave Lake for a family reunion. I was very nervous about how it would go, but I was excited for Casey as this would be her first camping trip.

We didn't bring my cane, but we did bring the stroller, in case I felt I needed it. But I actually didn't end up using it at all. I knew that the more I walked, the better I would get at it.

Walking back and forth between campsites was hard, and a few times I had to stop to take a break. It was only a minute or two's walk, but even that was extremely difficult, because of the uneven ground. My ankles were the weakest part of my legs, and they just weren't strong enough to allow me to go at a normal pace.

The weekend was fun and relaxing, and we played games, had some drinks, and just really enjoyed being around family. Although so much of my life was getting back to normal, one thing I noticed was just how tired I constantly was. All this walking I was doing now was taking a lot out of me. And as much as I wanted to stay up with everyone, I just couldn't, and I found myself in bed quite early both nights.

Casey had a blast camping, and now that she was sitting up, it was nice to be able to just plop her up on a blanket in the grass. She had no problem sleeping in the tent with us, although the mosquitoes were so bad that she ended up with quite a few bites. Of course, Casey didn't even seem to notice; she was her normal, happy self the entire time.

Unfortunately, once again, the weather hadn't been what we had hoped for. One of the days was sunny but very chilly, and the other was cloudy with rain on and off. I was really hoping to get a tan that weekend.

When we got home, James and I booked our flights to Phoenix. The summer was half over, and there really hadn't been many nice days. All our trips so far this summer had been disappointing weather-wise. All I wanted was to enjoy some sunshine. Booking our trip really gave me something to look forward to, for I knew that it would be nothing but sunshine in Phoenix!

We got some great deals on flights, and we booked for three weeks; my mom would join us for the first week. Having her there to help with Casey would be really nice. I had learned of a GBS Conference being held in the city on September 17, and I really wanted to attend, so we booked our flights for the following day.

On August 15, my mom, Casey, and I returned to the hospital. It was my first visit to the ICU in over two months. I had wanted to visit many times this summer, but I was determined not to return there until I knew I could walk in all by myself. And I finally felt that I was ready.

Upon walking into the unit, I felt strange. First of all, there was a strong "hospital smell" to it, although when I was a patient I had never once noticed it.

As I walked by the hospital rooms, I couldn't help but peek in at the patients lying in their beds. It was the ICU. Each and everyone here was in serious condition, and it made me feel sick to my stomach, thinking about what they were going through. I remembered what it felt like to be a patient in the ICU very well. It was the scariest experience of my life, and I could now admit that though sometimes I acted strong, I had actually been hoping I would just die, almost every minute of every day.

When we walked up toward the nurse's station, they all looked at me, having no idea who I was. They looked at Casey and then at my mom, and it was then that they realized who we were. The nurses barely recognized me or Casey, for that matter. My mom was the only one that looked the same, and she was the only reason why they realized who we all were.

All the nurses came over to see us, and they really couldn't believe how amazing I looked. I must have looked like a completely different person. And though I was still fairly slow, they were all beyond proud that I was walking again. I knew that seeing a patient that they had all cared for day after day, finally walking after months of being paralyzed, must have been very rewarding for them.

We also visited the other ward I had been on, and they as well couldn't have been happier or prouder of my improvement. I'm sure they knew that they had a huge role in my recovery, but actually seeing me walking must have really confirmed just how much.

Although I had thought it might be hard to go back to the hospital that day, it wasn't at all. It was actually a very joyful experience. I was happy to show them all that I had finally gotten my life back. It was great to see everyone again, most of all to be able to express my gratitude for the amazing care and treatment I had received there.

My walking continued to improve, and every week I could walk a little faster, a little longer, and with less pain. We tried to get out as much as possible, but due to me not having as much energy as before, we spent most of the last weeks of summer in the backyard with Casey.

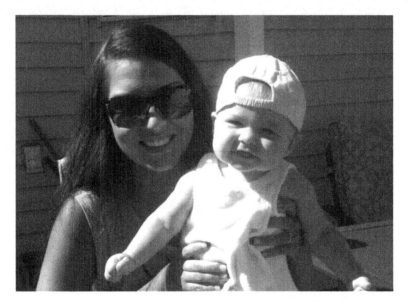

Casey and me

I was still so hot all the time, and I lived in shorts and a tank top the majority of the summer. I slept with a fan directly on me, which really helped at night, so I could at least sleep with a sheet. My feet were still extremely sensitive, and I found that even the cotton sheet caused me much pain while I slept. So I started sleeping with my feet hanging off the bed so that nothing would rub against my feet.

My legs were way stronger now than they had been during the previous month, and I could now finally bend down and pick up my daughter. I was also starting to be able to help with chores around the house, such as sweeping and tidying up.

The best part of my legs strengthening was that I could now shower while standing and didn't have to use the bath seat anymore. I was finally strong enough to stand for more than a few seconds; I was still lacking balance, though, so I would keep one hand on the wall for support. I kept the bath chair for a week or so just in case, but by the end of August, I was confident that I no longer needed it. So along with the bath seat, we also took back the toilet raiser, the wheelchair, and the walker. Taking all the equipment back was such a huge relief. My life was completely equipment-free.

September

At the beginning of the month, my brother proposed to his girlfriend. Our family couldn't have been happier for the two of them. With the first half of the year being so tough on us all, it felt really nice that good things were finally happening again. And now I had a wedding to look forward to!

My brother had proposed on a passenger bridge in the River Valley, and James suggested that we go for a walk and check it out since we had never been there before. I had been walking on my own for over a month, but I hadn't officially gone for a walk yet. For the most part, I only had to walk for very short distances, so I was intrigued to see how far I would be able to go.

The weather had been pretty cool during the last few days, so I wore jeans and a long-sleeve shirt. But the second we got to the River Valley and out of the car, I regretted it. Not only was the sun beaming down on us, but as soon as we started walking, I knew it was going to take a lot of work, and I was going to get really hot.

We walked for about five minutes to the bridge, and I was just sweating. It was crazy to me that a five-minute walk felt like a ten-minute run to me. We hung out there for a few minutes, checked out the view, and took some pictures. Then we turned around and headed back toward the car.

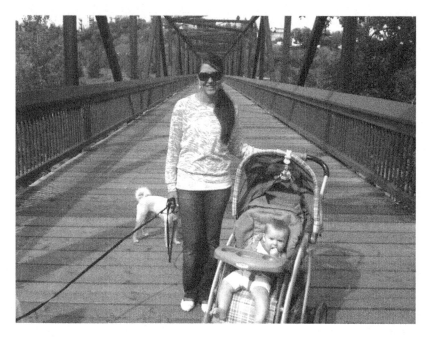

Me and Casey on my first real walk

When we got closer to the car, James asked if I could keep going onto another path. I said no. I knew he was disappointed; we had barely walked ten minutes, and I knew he could have walked all afternoon, but I just couldn't go any further. Not only was I very winded, hot, and tired, but also my ankles were starting to throb and ache. When my legs were really tired, they would start to buckle, and I risked falling. So we headed home.

Before I knew it, it was the day of the GBS Conference, September 17. Time was flying by for me, and I couldn't believe that it was nearly three months since I'd been released from the hospital.

At the conference, I ran into several familiar faces. First off, I ran into the woman with GBS, who had visited me when I was first admitted into the ICU. It was funny because I barely remembered her being at the hospital that day; it was quite a blurry memory in my mind, but as soon as I saw her, I remembered who she was. I even remembered some of the things we had talked about.

The man who had GBS and who had visited me throughout my time in the hospital was there along with his wife. I always loved talking with them. Although everyone's experiences with GBS are different, his journey was so similar to mine that I always went to him with any questions I had about my recovery.

I also ran into the young woman whom I had met just before I was transferred to the rehabilitation hospital. The last time I saw her, we were both in wheelchairs and she had yet to even try walking. She was now up walking with a walker. And for the first time, the shoe was on the other foot, and I felt a sense of pride for someone else's accomplishment. I remembered what it was like to get out of that wheelchair, and I was happy for her. She was also happy for me now that I was walking on my own, and I could tell that she was eager to get there too. I was happy to assure her that it would only be a matter of time.

It was very interesting to talk with other people who had suffered from GBS and to hear about their experiences. Everyone's stories were completely different. Some had it come on very quickly, like me, and were admitted to the hospital very quickly, while in other cases, it had taken days, even weeks, before they needed to be hospitalized Out of the large group of GBS survivors, there were only a few of us that had been put on a ventilator. Some people were only paralyzed from the waist down. Everyone had different struggles; some dealt with more pain, whereas others dealt with more fatigue. One common thing was that a lot of these people were still using things to help them walk, like canes, walkers, and even wheelchairs.

It became very apparent to me just how lucky I had really been. Yes, I had the worst possible case of GBS in the beginning; I was completely paralyzed from the neck down, had to be put on a breathing tube, and it had taken over six weeks for me to hit my plateau (when the normal time period is only two to three weeks.) But there weren't many people that had recovered as quickly as I did. Most of the people I met could not believe that I had only been out of the hospital for a few months. Some of these people were still recovering, and it had been years.

My neurologist was also there at the conference, and I'm sure he was surprised to see me walking around on my own. He was the one that had told me that it was unlikely I would walk for at least two years, and I was more than proud to show off that I had proved him wrong and had walked in less than five months.

When I reminded him that he had told me that, he said that it was always preferable to give patients the worst possible news, so that they could prepare for the worst possible scenario. But he reminded me that, keeping in mind the severity of my case, I had improved faster than his expectations. Usually, the longer it takes a patient to reach their plateau, the longer it takes for them to recover completely. This was definitely not the case with me. I was extremely lucky to have recovered as fast as I did, and it really could have been a lot worse than it was.

The following morning was September 18, which meant we were going to Phoenix! We were at the airport by 6:00 a.m., and I could not wait to start our vacation. The past year had been extremely challenging, both physically and mentally, and I was really looking forward to just relaxing by the pool with my family.

I wasn't sure how our almost eight-month-old would do on the flight, but we really should have known that, as always, she would be amazing. She couldn't have been any happier. She loved being around people so much that she just rested in our arms staring, smiling, and giggling at everyone around her. There were quite a few other babies on the flight; all were crying, and you could see in Casey's eyes that she was so concerned for them. She was such a good girl.

When we got to Phoenix, the weather was, of course, hot. Finally! As we made our way through the airport, I couldn't believe how big it was. By the time we got to our bags, then across the airport to the shuttle, and then over to the car rental, my feet were just aching, and I felt like I was going to faint. I tried to make my feet go faster, but they wouldn't, and I could not keep up with James and my mom. My ankles were so weak that I just couldn't walk as fast as a normal person.

I hadn't used my cane in over a month, but maybe I should have brought it for times like these, when I would be walking for long distances. It sure would have made the walk a lot easier.

We made the half-hour drive outside Phoenix to Gold Canyon. The home was in a gated community, nestling at the foot of the Superstition Mountains. James and I had never been to Arizona before; although we had both been to Vegas, we were right in the city, so we didn't get to see any of the countryside. The scenery was so different from the one at home or the tropical places we'd traveled to before. Seeing the Arizona desert, the red mountains, and the cacti everywhere was an incredibly beautiful experience.

When we got to the house in Gold Canyon, we couldn't believe our eyes. The home was absolutely stunning. It was paradise. It was a massive four-bedroom home, with a gorgeous pool in the back. I had known, without a doubt, that we were going to have an unbelievable time here.

The first day we spent lying by the pool, sunbathing, and sipping cocktails. I could definitely get used to this. But we also wanted to check out as much of the city while my mom was there to help with Casey. So the rest of our first week was very busy.

The second day we went to the zoo, and, thank god, they had a trolley tour to check out all the animals. After walking for about fifteen minutes, I just couldn't walk anymore, and if there hadn't been the trolley, I wouldn't have been able to continue with the rest of the zoo.

James especially wanted to golf, so he and I went in the afternoon while my mom stayed at the pool with Casey. That was, of course, the hottest day. Even with the cart, I had to stop after nine holes; my feet were aching badly, and I was just too exhausted to carry on.

On September 20, James and I left Casey with my mom, rented a convertible car, and drove up to the Grand Canyon for a helicopter tour. This was how we would celebrate our second wedding anniversary together. We had wanted to do so many different things on our first anniversary, but with me being five months pregnant, we didn't end up doing much. So this year, especially because of everything I had gone through, I wanted to do something extra special.

The drive up there was beautiful and also very fascinating. Although it was only a few hours away, the scenery changed drastically. Leaving Phoenix, it was over thirty-five degrees, and we were surrounded by desert and cacti. Then we started to get into the rolling hills, where you could see for miles and miles. As we got closer to the Grand Canyon, the weather dropped nearly fifteen degrees. The scenery was now thick forest, and it reminded me of the drive to Hinton, just before you get to the mountains in Alberta.

The helicopter tour over the Grand Canyon truly was one of the most unbelievable things I'd ever seen. We flew about ten minutes over the thick forest and then, all of a sudden, the trees just stopped, and it dropped off into the Canyon. I got to sit in the front with the pilot, and the floor underneath me was glass, which made it even more amazing. The Grand Canyon is not something you can easily describe, so I took a ton of pictures, but looking back on them, they really don't do it any justice. It was something James and I had always wanted to do, and we were happy to cross this off our bucket list.

We were going to stay overnight at a hotel, but decided that since it was only a few hours' drive back, we would rather just stay in the beautiful home we had back in Phoenix for free. I still felt like I was making up for lost time with my daughter and wanted to be with her as much as possible. So we drove back that evening.

I was especially excited to shop in Scottsdale one day and then in Mesa the next day. Although we did get some great deals and I bought several new pairs of flats, I was extremely frustrated that I couldn't shop as long as I wanted to. If I had been my old self, I could have shopped all day, but after only about half an hour and only a few stores, we had to leave because I was in too much pain.

The last few days that my mom was there, we checked out an aquarium and then an old Western Ghost Town, which were both very cool and luckily only involved a little bit of walking. The rest of the time, we spent relaxing by the pool, enjoying the sunshine. And before we knew it, our first week was over, and my mom was heading back to Edmonton. It wasn't that we didn't enjoy having my mom there; we certainly appreciated all the help with Casey, but we were looking forward to some family time, just the three of us.

On our first day, with just the three of us, Casey got her first cold. She was so stuffed up, and it broke my heart to hear her struggling to breathe when she slept. It certainly didn't affect her attitude, though; she was still her happy self, and she even started army crawling for the first time ever.

The second week wasn't as busy as the first, and I was quite happy to stay at the house by the pool day after day. I definitely wanted to get a nice tan. But in order to not get too bored, one of the days, we headed out to Canyon Lake. It was a beautiful lake right in the middle of the mountains, about twenty minutes away.

We rented a boat for an hour and had lunch out on the lake. Casey had to wear a life jacket, which she hated at first. But when she got to sit with her daddy while he drove the boat, she started to cheer up.

About halfway through our trip, I ran out of my medication. I wasn't used to going on a vacation with daily pills, and I hadn't even realized that I would need a refill before our trip was over. But a part of me wanted to see if I could go without them, so I didn't call for a prescription to be sent over.

Aside from the pain I got when I walked too far, I didn't have any neuropathic pain during the day, even without my pills. But at night, my feet ached so badly. I had a lot of trouble falling asleep that last week.

October

Another thing we wanted to do while in Phoenix was check out an NFL game. James is a huge NFL fan, and it had always been his dream to go to a game. A friend of ours told us to buy our tickets off a scalper, which was legal there and would be a lot cheaper.

Once we were parked, we walked by all the tailgate parties, which were unbelievable. Thousands of people were barbecuing with TVs and radios, so they could listen to the game right from the parking lot.

When we realized how far the walk was to where the scalpers were, James just left Casey and me waiting by the front doors. That way, I didn't have to walk anymore than I already had. And like our friends had told us, we got an amazing deal on seats in the tenth row.

Casey absolutely loved the game. It was so loud in there, which she thought was so much fun. She loved to be around people and was in her glory the whole time. Everyone around us couldn't help but smile and laugh as she giggled at anyone who would look at her. She sat in our arms looking around the stadium the entire game until the very end of it, when she fell asleep in our arms. Everyone was so amazed that she could fall asleep with all the noise going on around her.

During our last week in Phoenix, we surprisingly started to get bored. We felt that we had done everything we could do with a baby, and all we really had left to do was relax by the pool. I could certainly read magazines and tan all day long, but it actually started to cool down, so even that wasn't as enjoyable.

James really wanted to go hiking, and I felt really bad that unless he went on his own, he couldn't go. I could barely walk in a mall, let alone go for a hike. And I knew he wasn't comfortable going for a hike in the middle of the desert by himself.

Near the end of our trip, one of my respiratory therapists from the hospital e-mailed me. She also had a vacation home in Gold Canyon and was in town for a few days, so we headed there for lunch.

We spent the afternoon there, along with a few of their friends, and it was really nice to be around other people. James and I were certainly having an amazing time on our trip, but we were definitely missing our friends. On every other vacation we had gone on, we had either been with friends or we had met other couples. Since we weren't on a resort, we hadn't met anyone here. And three weeks was certainly a long time to go without hanging out with anyone else.

And the best part was that the respiratory therapist's husband also wanted to go for a hike, so he and James were able to get out on our last night in Phoenix.

After an amazing three weeks, our trip came to an end. I absolutely loved Phoenix; the weather had been beautiful, and we got to do so many fun things, in spite of my disability.

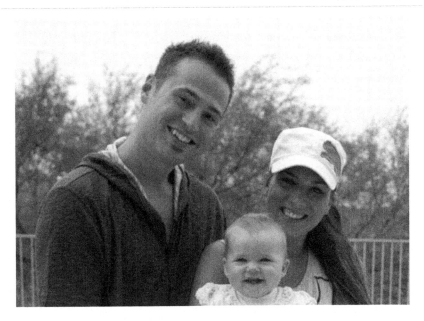

James, Casey and me in Phoenix

After returning the rental car, walking through the airport, and boarding our plane, I was so happy to realize that I wasn't as sore as I was the last time. I had walked the same distance through the airport just three weeks before and could barely do it, but now I could. I'm sure any sort of walking I had done on this trip had really helped strengthen my ankles.

Our first weekend back at home, we attended our friend's wedding reception. There was no way my ankles were strong enough to wear high heels, so I wore one of my several new pairs of flats that I had bought in Phoenix. It was really strange for me to not wear heels on a night out, though, and I was quite disappointed over it.

But this was the first time that I could actually dance. And I danced the entire night. My legs had never been strong enough to dance before, but now they were, so I took advantage of it and spent the entire night on the dance floor. I sure felt it the following morning; every part of my body ached from all the moving I had done.

On October 10, James headed back to work. His paternity leave was up, and fortunately, he was feeling comfortable enough to leave me at home. I felt confident that I could start taking care of myself and Casey.

I finally got my chance to be a stay-at-home mom with my daughter. She was eight months old, and I felt like I was now starting my maternity leave with her. I couldn't wait to have some alone time with her and do some mommy-daughter things together. I still couldn't drive a car, so we had to make do with being at home.

One of the first few things we did was go sit outside and play in the leaves. Watching her throw them up in the air over and over again and laughing her head off was priceless. It was so neat to watch her learning new things. And not just learning, but having such a great time doing it.

Over the next few weeks, Casey and I really started to bond. I was finally able to make her smile and laugh on command, and she was starting to reach her hands in the air to be picked up by me, which warmed my heart.

One evening, while going through bins of Casey's clothes for when she was older, I came across a knit sweater that looked familiar. I looked at James, and he said that I had picked that out for Casey one day at the hospital on one of the many trips to the lobby in my chair. I couldn't believe it. I thought I had dreamed about that. I vaguely remembered the sweater, but I didn't have any recollection of having James buy it for her.

On October 24, I went for a road test, which I passed, and I was reissued my driver's license. This was such a huge step in getting my independence back. Being stuck in the house all the time, unless I had someone to drive me places, was challenging, so I was so happy that Casey and I were no longer restricted to staying at home.

Casey and I started getting out and visiting with friends a lot more during the week. On weekends, I found myself leaving Casey with James and taking off to the mall to do some shopping. I was thrilled that I could finally get out all on my own, and I knew that the more I walked, the better it would be for me. It was then that I realized just how lucky I was that James and Casey were as close as they were. James was comfortable with her, even more than I was, since he had been raising her since birth. I was really happy that I could leave her with him and never have to worry about how she was doing.

At the end of October, I had an appointment with my neurologist. He wanted to assess my progress, as well as do an EMG test to test the activity levels in my leg muscles. I was not looking forward to it; the test would basically be electrocuting my legs.

But when my doctor came in to see me, he decided not to do the EMG. I was happy. He felt that he could plainly see how far my legs had come and that I was recovering very nicely. If something seemed to be recovering at a slower rate, then he would do the test to see where the problem was, but there was no reason to do it now. So he would just do an assessment.

Although I had definitely improved tremendously, the assessment showed that the left side of my body was still a lot weaker than my right. And overall, I was still not a hundred percent. I could barely stand on one leg; my balance was terrible. My ankles were also still weak. My doctor suggested that I try Yoga. It would really help with my balance and also strengthen my ankles and leg muscles.

On October 31, I started gentle yoga. I really surprised myself and found that I could actually do most of the exercises. The only ones that were really hard were the ones that involved me being up on my toes. My ankles just weren't strong enough for me to go onto my toes yet. With my balance being so bad, I also found I had to hold onto the wall for balance with some exercises.

November

I continued getting stronger and stronger, especially from the yoga I was doing. But I wasn't back to normal yet, even if I looked like I was.

The pain in my feet was actually getting worse. The sensitivity was getting stronger, and even the smallest touch hurt so badly. The aches and shooting pains in them at night were at their worst, and I struggled to fall asleep every night. My energy level was nowhere near what I used to have; not only was I sleeping ten hours a night, but I also needed to nap for a few hours every day. Luckily, Casey was still napping twice a day, so I had that chance.

My voice was still so scratchy and hoarse that people constantly asked me if I was sick. The interesting thing was that my throat actually did feel sore, as if I had a cold, but only when I talked. I assumed it was my vocal cords that were causing me the discomfort.

I was still hot all the time, although with the weather getting colder, it was getting better. Thankfully, I could finally use my straightener again without feeling like I was going to faint.

November 19 was my twenty-seventh birthday. This was a very special day for me. Although most people dread getting older, I was thrilled as this meant I was still alive. I was grateful that I had made it to my birthday this year. And even more grateful that I could finally curl my hair again!

Many of my friends came out that night; we were all getting older and barely went out anymore, so I was amazed at the number of people that showed up. We hung out at our place for a bit and then headed to a new pub downtown for drinks.

After one drink too many, while talking to my girlfriends about everything I had gone through, I started bawling about my scar. I had come to terms with most of the scars on my body, except for the one on my neck. I felt that it was the first thing people saw when they saw me, and I hated that so much. My girlfriends assured me that I was beautiful no matter what. And being around all my friends and family that evening showed me just how lucky I was to have all these amazing people in my life. The scar really wasn't important.

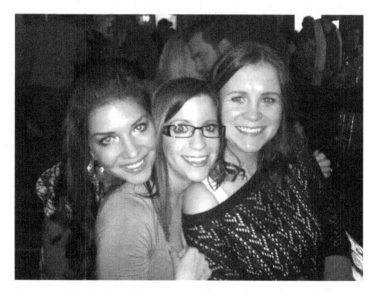

With friends on my birthday

I found myself back visiting the ICU again; we had forgotten a few things at the house in Phoenix, so my RT had brought them into his office for me to pick up. It was always nice to see those who had helped me in the hospital, especially the ones that weren't on shift the last time I was there. I knew they all especially loved seeing Casey and how much she had grown.

By the end of November, I was so impressed with how much yoga was helping me. I could actually stand on my tippy toes now, and my balance was way better than it had been just a few weeks before. Like always, I was getting better and better all the time.

December

My energy level was still pretty low, and I was still sleeping a lot, but for the first time, I no longer felt limited by my walking. When I went to the mall or for walks, although I could feel my ankles working harder, they didn't get sore anymore. I could finally keep up with everyone around me. I used to have limits and could only walk for a certain amount of time, but now I never felt like I couldn't keep going.

It finally looked like I might be ready to return to work. My insurance company wanted to see when I would be ready and sent me for a physiotherapy assessment. The physiotherapists would assess me and then recommend a date for me to return. They would also advise on any problems or limitations I would have at work, as well as recommend exercises to help fix these problems.

It was quite interesting seeing new physiotherapists. They knew that I had GBS and that my muscles would be weaker than those of the normal person. They knew how serious it had been, and they knew how quickly I had recovered. But that's not what they were looking at today. The focus of most of the PTs I had seen up until now had been to compare me with how I had done on the last assessment. But these PTs were comparing me strictly with a normal person.

They tested my strength, which had definitely improved from yoga, but my ankles were still very weak. I still had a lot of trouble squatting. When the PT asked me to walk across the room so he could see my walking, he mentioned to his coworker that my walking was really bad. I basically walked flat-footed.

I hadn't really noticed it before but now that he mentioned it, I realized that when I walked, I didn't lift my toes up. I stepped with my entire foot and placed it flat on the ground, instead of placing my heel and then my toes down. My feet would slap down on the ground, creating a loud flopping sound. My ankles weren't strong enough to lift the front of my foot up. And they weren't strong enough because I wasn't lifting my toes up. It was a vicious circle.

After my assessment, the physiotherpists recommended that I complete eight weeks of therapy with them. I had improved a lot, but I was not back to one hundred percent yet. I could certainly do my job again, and I could probably do the majority of the things in my life that I had done before. But their job was to get me back to one hundred percent and ensure that I could do everything I did before my illness. Plus, they were concerned with how sitting for eight hours a day, could affect my muscles. They knew that they still needed a lot more work, and sitting would not be good for them.

It was halfway through December, and with the Christmas holidays coming up, on top of the wait to get in, I would be starting my eight weeks of therapy at the end of January.

A lot of my friends were shocked to hear that I needed to go back for more physiotherapy and assumed that I was disappointed about the setback. But I wasn't at all; it was quite the opposite. I didn't see it as a setback at all; I saw it as a way to continue improving myself. I still couldn't even stand in a pair of heels, let alone walk in them, so getting back to wearing them was one of my main priorities. I had jogged to the mailbox once, and it was so hard that I wanted to learn how to run again. It's not like I ran often before my illness, but I at least wanted to have the option. I certainly didn't want to be limited to running after Casey because I physically couldn't do it.

The assessment was an eye-opener, and I realized that if I wanted my legs to get stronger, I would have to do more about it. Since I was still more than a month away from starting my physiotherapy, I decided to start working out at home and strengthening them on my own. And although the first few weeks were hard, it got easier and easier each time I did it.

Christmas was extra special this year. Of course, it was partly because of my newfound appreciation for life, but it was also Casey's first Christmas. And even though she didn't understand what was going on, it was still such a joy to watch her open her presents and get a whole bunch of new toys to play with. I was so thankful that I was there to share her first Christmas with her.

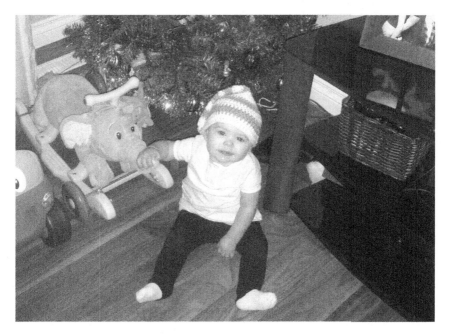

Casey at Christmas time

January 2012

The pain in my feet was still extremely annoying; they were tingly and sensitive during the day and throbbing at nighttime. I assumed that it was something I just needed to live with, but I ended up talking to my doctor about it because it was starting to really affect my sleep.

He informed me that the dosage I was on for my medication was very low, so he would simply increase it. And once the dosage was changed, I immediately noticed a difference. My feet still tingled and throbbed a bit, but not nearly as bad as before, and I could finally fall asleep at night.

Another positive thing that I noticed one day was that my hair was finally growing back! I had small pieces of hair that were peeking throughout my head. And as the days went on, the pieces of hair grew longer and longer. When I saw all the short pieces of hair I had, I realized just how much had actually fallen out.

On January 21, I started attending a GBS Support Group. I had met several people at the conference who were interested in meeting every few months, and I knew that it would be a great place to not only have questions answered, but also to just be around other people that had experienced GBS. With it being such a rare disease, there weren't many people that could relate to me.

Being at the meeting that day was yet another eye-opener. There were about eleven of us there. I had met most of them at the conference back in September, but getting to talk to them more really showed me how lucky I had been. Many of them were still dealing with weakness in their legs, and some of them were still in wheelchairs. They were all still dealing with symptoms, even though it had been years for some of them. I definitely felt for them. I knew I wasn't one hundred percent yet, but I was pretty darned close.

On January 23, I started physio three days a week. It was more like going to the gym. They gave me a binder full of exercises to work specific parts of my body that I needed to strengthen, and I would go at it on my own.

I started out by walking on the treadmill for ten minutes at a time. Each class, I increased my walking more and more until I was up to thirty minutes. Then I increased my pace. I spent the rest of my two-hour session doing squats, lunges, and various strengthening exercises. Every few classes, I increased the weight or the amount of repetitions I did.

January 26 was Casey's first birthday. Once again, I was grateful that I was alive to share it with her. We had our closest friends and family over, and she opened her presents, ate cake, and played with her friends. I noticed that bending down and squatting was getting easier as I had done a lot of it that afternoon.

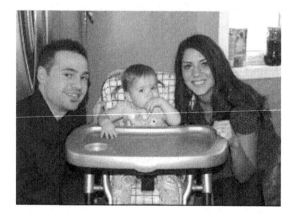

James and me with Casey on her first birthday

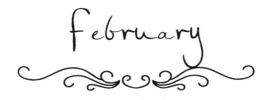

February

I could not believe that it had been six months since my best friend had been home from working on the cruise ship. We picked up right where we had left things half a year earlier, and it was so great to have her home again. I told her about my physio and about how I still couldn't wear high heels or run. She reminded me that the last time she saw me, I was just starting to walk with a cane. In her eyes, I was doing amazing.

Casey was a flower girl in one of our best friends' wedding on February 18. We had hoped that she might be walking by now, but she wasn't, so I pulled her down the aisle in a sled. I was so nervous about walking down that aisle; I knew that my walking was fine now, but who knew how I would do under pressure. I was wearing flats, but I was still scared that I would fall on my face in front of everyone. I did perfectly fine, though, and besides, everyone's eyes were on my beautiful daughter all dressed up sitting in the sled.

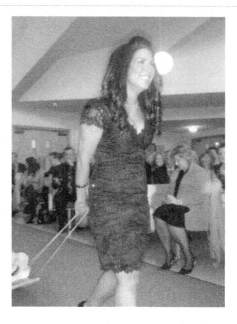

Walking down the aisle at a friend's wedding

In physio that week, I started running on the treadmill. It was very strange at first, and the impact from my feet hitting the treadmill was very painful. I could only run for a minute before my ankles would start aching and I would have to slow down. So I ran for one minute and then walked for two for thirty minutes.

My PTs assessed me again to see how much I had improved in the past month, and we were all very pleased with my progress. I had increased my weights drastically, and I was lifting more than I could even before I was in the hospital. My ankles were still weak, though definitely stronger than before, but they were getting better from running.

February 22 marked my one-year anniversary of being admitted to the hospital. What a year it had been. I had given birth to my first child and then spent four extremely difficult months in the hospital. But it was all behind me now. I had improved so much, and it really was remarkable how far I'd come. The doctors had told me that I might not walk for two years, and here I was, running.

fast forward

I'm grateful to be back home with my daughter again. Casey and I are very close now, and although it took a while, I actually feel like she loves me as much as her daddy now. But I do know that one of the best things to come from this whole experience is the bond it created between Casey and James. They now have an unbelievable connection from the time they spent with one another. I'm so happy that they had that time together as most men don't ever get that with their children. And anyone who knows them can see it in their eyes just how much love they have for one another.

Casey has now started walking. Seeing her place her feet one foot in front of another, while trying to keep her balance, has been absolutely amazing to me. Any other person might look at her and think nothing of it; she is just doing what babies do. But I don't.

Since she took her first steps, she has improved every day, and I am amazed by her. I remember what it was like to learn how to walk again. It was anything but easy, and I had over twenty-six years of practice behind me. She is learning completely from scratch.

I remember all the times I wanted to give up on walking. Seeing Casey get right back up every time she falls, with a huge smile on her face, has shown me just how determined my little girl is. I know exactly what she is going through, and I am proud of all her hard work.

I know that every step she takes is strengthening her little legs and ankles, which will make it easier for her to eventually run her little heart out. And because of my hard work, I will be right behind her, running after her.

I've since finished physio, and I couldn't be any happier for having gone through the program. I remember going in thinking that there wasn't much I needed to work on, but I really have improved so much in such a short time. Since finishing physio, I have even started walking in high heels for short periods.

In mid March, I headed back to work. I started working only a few hours a day, a few days a week, and gradually increased my hours each week. Going back to work was the last step to getting my life back. It feels great to be back at my career again, and my life really does feel back to normal. In August, I even landed my dream job, only a few minutes away from our home.

Since finishing physio, I've also started running outside. Running in physio strengthened my ankles so much so I know I need to continue with it. I am now running four kilometres, doing intervals of running one minute and walking for forty-five seconds. Although that's all my ankles can handle as this point, I know that I will only get better.

Although on the outside I may look like I have recovered completely, there are still a lot of things that are difficult for me, like getting out of the bath and getting up off the floor. I have to get on all fours before I can get up, just like they taught me back at the rehabilitation hospital. There is no way I can push off on my ankles without help from my arms. With my balance being nowhere where it should be, I still can't stand on one leg without falling over. I put my pants and shoes on while leaning against a wall, and I often lose my balance when walking- especially when wearing high heels, or when walking on uneven ground.

I do walk at a normal pace again, but I have to think about every single step I make. The muscles in my feet are still weak, so I have to be sure that I place my foot in a specific way to ensure that I don't twist my ankle. I also still suffer from foot drop, and my toes quite often catch the ground when I walk.

I think the worst of my residual symptoms are the aches I have in my muscles. After twenty minutes of sitting, every time I stand, my muscles are tight and my whole body is extremely sore. It takes a few minutes to stretch out my muscles. By the end of the day, my legs ache and cramp up, like I ran for hours and hours. I constantly feel sore, and I often feel like I'm eighty years old.

My feet are still numb and tingly and very sensitive, to the point where the tiniest pebbles feel like glass on my feet. I'm not sure that will ever go away. But if these are my residual symptoms, I can definitely deal with them. I know that things could certainly have been a lot worse.

My missing chunks of hair have grown out about four inches now, and I will eventually have my thick head of hair back. After all this time, my voice has actually improved a little over the last few months. I know it's definitely not the same as it was before GBS; I can't sing those high notes without my voice cracking, but everytime I see my girlfriend from out of town, she comments that she's noticed an improvement.

My scars will always be there; it's something that I've learned to accept. And although I may not like them, I am no longer ashamed of them. They remind me every day of what I have gone through. And now that they are all healed, they just symbolize that everything I went through is all over with and in the past.

When I look back on my time in the hospital, it's almost hard to believe that I even went through everything I did. Sometimes, I will hear a song, like *The Climb* by Miley Cyrus, or experience a smell, like the body wash the nurses used for my sponge baths, which will remind me of being back in that hospital bed. And it truly makes me want to cry. My memories are fuzzy, and there's so much that I don't remember, but I do remember the knot I felt in my stomach. It felt like I was having an anxiety attack for three straight months. I felt like I was in a nightmare that I just couldn't wake up from.

I will always remember the nausea, the puking, and the pain that I went through every single day. I will always remember that I wanted to give up so many times, and I remember begging my family day after day to just let me die. And if I hadn't been paralyzed, I probably would have ripped out my breathing tube, and who knows if I would still be here today. Everyone told me that I would get better, but I never believed them until months later when I started to improve.

Looking back on those months I spent recovering, it's hard to even remember when I didn't have the strength to move my own body. I remember trying as hard as I could, using all my energy and force to move my toes, but I couldn't. I remember trying as hard as I could to turn on the TV and not being able to. I remember trying to hold a cup in my hand and not being able to. But I also remember the days when I finally could do it all. And that is an amazing feeling that I will always remember.

My journey with Guillain-Barré Syndrome was such a challenging experience, and my recovery seemed to take forever. But looking back at the last year has shown me that the speed with which I recovered was a miracle. Although at times it felt like it was taking forever, especially during those first months in the hospital, it actually went by extremely fast.

It's quite incredible what happened to me. Not everyone has to learn how to use every muscle in their body again. And I don't think I could ever be more proud of myself than I am now. I've definitely learned not to take life for granted anymore. Being completely healthy at twenty-six, my health had never really crossed my mind before. But after going through what I did, I truly realize just how special life really is.

Many times, I thought my life was over; I didn't think I would ever get to enjoy being a mother like I had always dreamed of. I'm so grateful to those who were there for me, and who told me over and over that things would eventually go back to the way they were.

I did get my life back, and I am finally able to live my life—Happily Ever After.

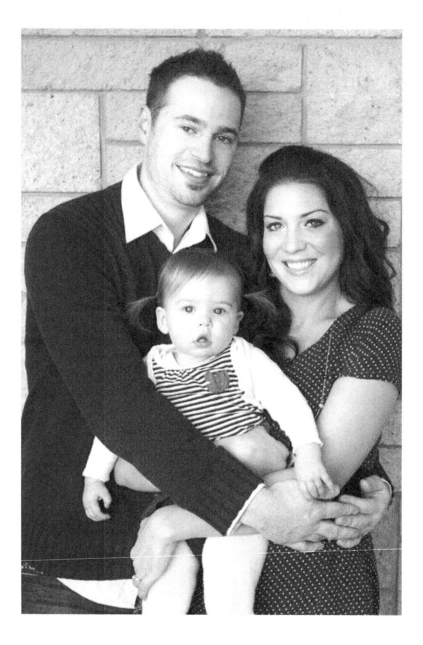

Made in the USA
Monee, IL
25 March 2021

63744823R00134